HOW TO FIGHT BREAST CANCER AND WIN!

A MATTER OF LIFE AND HEALTH

DEANN AKANDE, M.D.

ACKNOWLEDGEMENTS

This book is written in remembrance of my Mother, Margaret Robinson, who was a breast cancer survivor, my sister Karen, and to all who have been diagnosed with this disease and their family members. I hope that you will find this book a welcomed resource for you at this particular time. My wish for you is a cureor a remission from this dreaded disease and success at preventing disease or its recurrence in the future.

I give special consideration, thanks and love to my husband Isaac who has been with me through this fight. He has been a faithful prayer warrior and an encouragement for me from the very start.

CONTENTS

PREFACE

This book has been written for You. It is also written for your Mother, your Grandmother, your Sister, your Aunt, your Niece, your Cousin, your Friend or someone else you may know. It was not written just to sit on a book shelf. Take it and read it. It is a matter of life and health. Take the information in this book to heart and share the information in it with others. It just may save your life or the life of someone you know.

This is not just another book about breast cancer. The first part of this book is a record of my personal experience as a physician and a patient diagnosed with the disease of breast cancer before the age of 31 and again sixteen years later. The initial presentation of my breast cancer and the unusual presentation of the recurrence of breast cancer in my case I hope will give you better insight into this disease and make you more astute so that you will not dismiss minor changes in your breasts, which may need attention.

Every case of breast cancer is similar, but each case may be different in its presentation, stage ande grade of disease and cellular and subcellular or molecular features. Treatment plans may vary depending on the presentation of the disease, the tumor charateristics, the patient age, physical constitution, emotional needs and desires. This book will give you significant and understandable and usable information on breast cancer detection, diagnosis, conventional treatments for early breast cancer and treatment for cancer that has metastasized (spread outside the breast), treatment for the side effects of treatment, complementary alternative treatments, diet, nutrition and supplements and exercise. The Pathology Atlas which will familiarize you with the terminology in your Pathology Report.

Breast cancer is no longer a death sentence, when diagnosed early. It has become for many women who live with the disease, a chronic and treatable condition. Current treatment plans and earlier detection have lengthened disease free intervals. Vigilant surveillance is imperative once the disease is discovered. It is my hope for you that with the aid of this book you may transform and make meaningful lifestyle changes to either prevent breast cancer by either minimizing your risk for the disease. If you have had breast cancer I hope this book will aid you in minimizing the risk for disease recurrence.

As the title of this book implies, my intention is to empower the reader to be able to cope and fight breast cancer and win or to more simply put it this book is about how to overcome this deadly disease. As a physician (medical doctor) I understand that you would like to just go straight to the battle plan or treatment regimen to fight this disease.

I have even enclosed pathology pictures in this book in a loosely progressive order. My best suggestion of the use of these pictures to aid you in the understanding of the different types of breast cancer. if you cannot understand it by yourself, have your doctor or a physician friend or medical student explain it to you. I hope that by introducing these pictures to a doctor or a physician friend, will give you an opportunity to learn or to have an idea of what changes are caused in your breast by this disease. But I know that there are some book-worms out there that can understand these pictures by themselves. Nevertheless, I hope this book brings you closer to your doctor or physician friend to open up a dialogue between you to help educate you more about this disease while the pictures are being explained to you. If you do not have a doctor or physician or medical student friend who will explain this to you, don't worry your head about it. Just glance through the pictures and have an idea what is going on with cells in the breast.

Before we get to the battle plan or treatment regimen, the first parts or eleven chapters of this book tell my personal private encounter with this disease, as a thirty-one year old physician in the prime of her life. I have chosen to share these three chapters with you because the first encounter is always the toughest, because when you first hear the word cancer as a diagnosis you think of death. In those three chapters, you will see how I felt a mass in my left breast and even though I explained all the actions I took to get treatment very sanely in the first three chapters, at the time I felt as though I was in a whirlwind and being torn apart. I was afraid of losing my life in its prime. I am sure my lifestyle at the age of 31 will mimmicked the lifestyle of any young lady of my generation that just finished their college education and the foundation for their life. In my case, I had just finished twelve years of college education that included medical school and residency and was just about to start reaping the rewards of my education when this happened.

Again before getting to the battle plan and the treatment regimen for this disease, chapters 4 through 11 are my encounter with this disease the second time around. This disease this time around showed up as a mass under my right arm. Many people are not familiar with this underarm mass as being breast cancer, but most physicians do know. I knew better than to do the things I was doing, but I was in a state of denial and procrastinated until the pain I was experiencing was undeniable. My advice is that if you feel any pain in your upper arm or shoulder that refuses to go away, see you doctor. It may not be a pulled muscle, it might breast cancer that may be causing the symptoms. The second time around was more scary that the first time because the disease was now in lymph nodes which means it had spread outside the breast and was no longer confined. But thanks to age and maturity, I was more resolute that I would overcome the disease. I hope my account in chapters 4 to 11 will make a good reference as to how as a physician I went about coping with the treatment and I hope that by you having this treatment in mind, it could facilitate you in your treatment planning. In other words, you will have an idea of what treatment to expect during treatment and what to ask about.

Chapters 12 through 21 is the first part of the battle plan, the breast health primer that will familiarize you with your breast. The journey of a thousand miles started with the very first step. In this section of the book, you get to know the anatomy of your own breasts, breast care, breast health examination, knowing breast cancer risk factors, the mammogram, once you discover a mass what's next, benign conditions of the breasts (Any time a tumor is BENIGN it means non-cancerous). In this section, I have listed about nineteen benign conditions, borderline lesions and intraductal neoplasia (pre-cancerous and cancerous findings in the breast that are confined the to ducts in the breast and have not spread outside the ducts), and malignant neoplasms of the breast (Any time a tumor is MALIGNANT it is cancer. This is not good.) I have listed many of the most common types malignant neoplasms. Next is the pathology atlas. The atlas is a collection of the pathology pictures that I ask you to share with doctor or physician friend if you need them explained to you or if you need help to start a dialogue with your physician about your diagnosis of cancer. As I said earlier, if you don't have anyone to share with, just glance through it and have an idea what the cells of the breast look like.

Next is the breast cancer grading (Breast cancer grading is how a pathologist evaluates the tumor as to whether or not it is forming tubules or ducts, the grading of the nucleus of the tumor cells (what the nucleus size and shape and coarseness of the material in the nucleus looks like) and the mitoses (the number of cells that are dividing). Breast cancers are graded from low grade to high grade (I to III). The last part of the primer is the breast cancer staging. (This is how far a tumor has spread in the body, whether it has spreading to the brain, the liver or the bones or into the lymph nodes. This can be determined by radiological tests like X-rays, CT liver and bone scans, biopsies, the examination of the resected tumor and the simple clinical examination as performed by the pathologist. I will not bore you with all the classification of the staging.)

The surgical pathology report is then described. It includes the weighing, measuring and gross description of the breast tissue removed and the type of procedure from which the tissue was obtained. This may be from a needle core biopsies which are obtained when a needle is inserted into the suspected area of breast to sample and examine the tissue or mass to determine if it is cancerous or non-cancerous. The breast mass may also be surgically removed or excised (lumpectomy) or by removing a quadrant of the breast (quadrantectomy), by removal of the breast (mastectomy), by removal of the breast with lymph nodes or only a lymph node sampling only or sentinel node (closest lymph node to the breast under the arm) removal. The tissue removed by the surgeon is examined and slides as prepared and the cells are looked at under the microscope by the pathologist in order to determine whether or not the tissue is benign or malignant. If the tissue is malignant or cancerous, the histologic type of the tumor is determined as well as the grade of the tumor and adequacy of the margins of excision of the tumor. If the tissue is malignant other tests will be ordered by the pathologist which are necessary to further classify the cancer for treatment purposes.

A chapter on the current chemotherapy treatments is included, which lists side effects or adverse reactions of each drug. Radiation therapy after lumpectomy and mastectomy is discussed. There is also a chapter on breast reconstruction. Adjuvant treatments or treatments used besides chemotherapy and radiation therapy are discussed. There is an extensive chapter on palliative therapy or the treatment to reduce pain suffering, and the impact of disease and the side effects of treatment included which has a discussion on fever, nausea and vomiting, adjuvant hormonal therapy and menopausal symptoms, physical therapy, anxiety and depression and pain control. There is an extensive chapter on the risk reduction of breast cancer by nutrition and exercise. The Complementary alternative medicine (CAM) therapy chapter includes the following subjects: psychological therapy, support groups, nutritional supplements and herbal therapies, acupuncture, massage therapy, progressive muscle relaxation, stress relief, exercise after surgery, yoga, biotherapy and immunotherapy, spirituality and prayer. The last part of the book includes a personal breast cancer journal which you can use.

<u>Very Important Notice</u>

Please remember that this book is written by a breast cancer survivor who happens to be a medical doctor. Please bear with me as I am trying my best to explain medical terminologies in this book in the layman's language. I do not expect you to be able to understand every medical treatment aspect in this book, but I surely hope that it will embolden you to ask questions about your treatment in order to better understand what your physician is saying. Remember how when a doctor is explaining the condition of a patient to the patient's family and how when the doctor has finally finished talking in medical terms, someone always asks the doctor please can you now explain that in English (jokingly), that is in layman's terms? Therefore, if you are having any problems with aspects of the medical terms in this book do not hesitate to ask your doctor or physician friend. However, if you do not have a medical doctor or physician friend, I welcome your questions at <u>MDAkande@yahoo.com</u>. Do not hesitate to contact me.

If you know anyone who is fighting breast cancer right now, there is a companion Breast Cancer Journal for this book which can be used as a diary for patients to keep track of their treatments. They can compare their treatment with the treatments in this book. It is because of such people who are battling breast cancer right now that I have included my personal account or experience in the first eleven chapters of this book. At least when you or a loved one are going through treatment will have something to read to motivate them of how a physician who is familiar with such disease coped during treatment in order to avoid any sort of depression or self-defeatist attitude that is detrimental to helping the body in healing itself while receiving and coping with treatment regimen. I know when I was going through my chemotherapy treatments, I wish I had a book to read about how somebody else coped with the treatment.

However, if you are just reading this book for prevention or if you are a survivor already, that means that you are trying to enamor yourself. I will suggest that you have a reading meeting with a couple of your friends or daughters or sisters. Read the book together as a group and discuss past experiences and family histories either of one or of any in the group. By reading this book together with friends or family you will likely have certain medical terminologies explained amongst each other. I am hoping that you will have a nurse, a doctor or a health care professional in the group. If not I will suggest that you put on a pot of tea and plan a discussion get-together or meeting and invite into the group a nurse, a doctor or a health care professional. Again if you cannot find anyone to invite, leave me an email at the above address and we will set a time, hopefully on a weekend, so that I can join your group conversation by telephone.

My hope is to get women of all ages, those who have dealt with this disease and those who have not, friends, sisters, daughters and mothers to discuss and help each other defeat this dreaded disease if it dare attacks any of them. For I realize that by talking about it, reading about it and preparing yourself before you have to deal with it goes a long way in winning the battle, because it diminishes the fear which makes things worse. Again do not let the medical jargon bother you, I want it to actually encourage you to make friends with the nurse (who specializes in the treatment of this disease), a doctor or physician, preferably a friend or a health care worker familiar with cancer treatment. I strongly believe that it is a good thing for every friend group, or sister, mother and daughters group to have a health care professional in their clique. If you do not have one, recruit one, befriend one or adopt one. My point is that you cannot afford to only investigate this disease only during your normal doctor visits. It shouldn't be that the only time you can discuss this disease is when you get billed for it. But if that is what it takes to make you start a dialogue with your physician, then ask as many questions as you can about breast cancer prevention during you regular doctor visits. Make that paid time with you physician count. Go in with a list of questions, like it's a grocery list if you have trouble remembering what you what to ask. After all you are paying for the time. Remember all the free information that you got from your doctor or physician friend or nurse and bring them up during your regular doctor visit. The point is you should have a relationship with your doctor in which you can ask as many questions as you want to and take notes when it concerns your care. Remember, I want you to be an informed patient taking an active role in your treatment plans and care.

THE FIRST TIME AROUND

MY FIRST MAMMOGRAM

I was thirty-one years old, and lying on the bed when I thought that I felt a mass in my left breast. The next day I was examined by another physician. She told me that she did not feel a mass. She said that the only thing the she could feel was my ribs. I tried to feel the mass again, but only felt my ribs also and not a mass. It felt good to have her assurance that it was only my ribs. I guess that this is just part of the blessing of having dense slightly nodular breasts. She did not order a mammogram and I did not request one at that time, after all I was thirty-one years old and my yearly mammogram screenings will not begin until I'm thirty-five and by many physicians that would be considered early. My physician and I had agreed that I would start having yearly mammograms earlier since my mother had had breast cancer. I continued with my monthly self-examinations and I never felt any additional changes.

Three years later on a Thursday, a hot, sultry and blustery day in August at age thirty-four, I was sitting in my comfortable, climate controlled, air-conditioned office at the hospital with a little time on my hands. The surgical caseload had been light and none of the scheduled surgical cases would require the attention of a pathologist or my immediate consultation to the surgeon about the case. There were no tissue biopsies (biopsies or samplings of a mass) or frozen section (quick freezing of the tissue to be immediately examined by the pathologist) listed on the surgical schedule. I called the surgery department to see if there were any add-on cases or any changes in the schedule.

There were no changes so I felt safe to use the time to my advantage and schedule an appointment that afternoon for my first mammogram. I knew that I was scheduling a few months earlier than the recommended guidelines, but I decided to get it done while it is on my mind and while I had the time. I called Dr. Claudia's office and surprisingly she had an opening. I was in luck. There had been a cancellation of an appointment about an hour earlier, so I told them I would fill that slot. I informed my secretary as to where I would be for the next hour or so and that I would return promptly to complete the gross examination of the afternoon surgery specimens.

Dr. Claudia had been a classmate of mine from medical school.

This was the first time that I had ever been to her office. The office staff was quite congenial. I was given the usual barrage of paperwork to complete. You would think that they would know by now that the more forms a doctor has to fill out the less legible the handwriting becomes, after all it is common knowledge that physicians go to medical school to learn how to write like a doctor. I completed the paperwork and returned it to the assistant at the desk. I then returned to my seat in the waiting room. Five minutes later my name was called. I was taken to a room with blue and yellow   feminine country decor and color coordinated lockers. I was instructed to strip from the waste up, to remove my necklace and to put the drape over my upper torso. I was told that my personal removed items should be stored in the locker and that I should remove the key with the attached plastic yellow coil chain from the locker, place my clothes and belongings in the locker and put the key on my wrist. I did as I was instructed; stripping from the waist up and putting on the pink and blue flowered cotton drape and waited for my name to be called.

A technician called me. I accompanied her to the mammography room. She asked if I had any special problems with my breasts, any previous surgeries, or any first-degree relatives that had breast cancer. I told her that my mother had breast cancer and had lived some 26 years after the diagnosis and did not have a reoccurrence or die of the disease. I also advised her that my mother's grandmother had had breast cancer and that my father had a sister with breast cancer. The technician noted this on the history form. She also asked me whether or not I used any deodorant. I told her that I had but that it was not the type of deodorant that had aluminum chlorohydrate and or talc in it so wouldn't interfere with the procedure. I was allergic to the aluminum chlorohydrate and talc, most deodorants contain one or both of these ingredients.

I was then told to remove the cotton drape and the examination began. I was positioned in the mammography unit by the technician. The unit was a piece of equipment with a platform and a clear plastic rectangular plate on a slide used for compression of the breast. The technician stood behind a shield when the films were shot to prevent her exposure to the radiation. The procedure was quite painful for me. I felt that instead of the rectangular plastic plate being called a compressor, the device should more appropriately be called a breast smasher. If you have breasts that are big and voluptuous before the procedure, the breasts would definitely be flat and smashed after the procedure. If you have multiple cysts before the procedure, you undoubtedly will be cured and have none left after the procedure. I was relieved when the compression stopped. I reflected in silence that if men had to undergo this procedure, they would have invented a better method or procedure years ago. Most men would be intolerant to this kind of pain. What things we go through just because we're female!

After about forty-five minutes of examination, the technician took the films to Dr. Claudia. She later came back and said that Dr. Claudia wanted to see me. Claudia greeted me when I entered her office. We looked at the films together. We looked at the right breast films first and it was normal. We viewed the films of my left breast. I didn't like what I was seeing. I asked her, "Are you sure that these are my films?" She said, "Yes." The only thing that I could think about was that this is my first mammogram and it is malignant. The images of the right breast were normal, but the left breast had two areas of finely stippled calcifications(or white spots or densities on the x-ray film), both areas were located very close to the muscles of the chest wall by the ribs. The pattern of the left breast film or x-ray was unmistakable and indicative of malignancy or cancer. I couldn't cry. I had no time for tears. I just felt a rush deep inside of me and a sense of urgency that something must be done and that it needed to be done right now. Claudia asked me if there was any one that I wanted to call. I told her that I needed to call the plastic surgeon. I called Dr. JR, whom I knew during my residency. The one thing that I definitely knew was that I wanted to be reconstructed, after all I was only thirty-four years old, unmarried and had my whole life ahead of me.

When I called Dr. JRs office, his nurse answered the phone and stated that he was not in the office on Thursday afternoon and that it was his day off. She said that he usually plays tennis in the afternoon. Just as soon as she had completed her last sentence she said, "I can't believe my eyes! He just walked into the office and he never comes in on his day off! I asked her to please put him on the line. I asked Dr. JR why he came to his office on his day off and he told me that God told him to go to his office. I told him that I urgently needed to see him and that I was in Dr. Claudia's office. I was looking at my first mammogram. I told him that I needed to see him now. He told me to bring the films and to come over right now.

I thanked Claudia, hopped into my silver BMW with the films in hand and proceeded to see Dr. JR. I had no time for tears. I wondered what I may have found if I had a mammogram performed at age thirty-one when I thought that I had felt something. I thought about the times that I had been to see my gynecologist and that he had not performed a breast examination each time. I thought about the fact that I should requested my physician to order a mammogram when I first thought that I felt something in my breast even though she did not feel it and even though mammography was not recommended until age forty and my screening was scheduled earlier because of my family history. I should have had a mammogram at age thirty-one regardless of the protocols, because I was at high risk for the disease. I still couldn't feel anything now by palpation, not did I feel anything on my monthly breast self examinations. Who knows if I had anything that may have been visible on mammogram when I was thirty-one years old. I may or may not have found anything on mammography back then. This is now and that was then, I only had the determination that this disease was not going to kill me.

I reflected on the day when I arrived home from college for the Thanksgiving holiday and my Dad informed me that my Mom had a mass in her right breast about the size of a hen's egg and that he couldn't get her to go to the doctor to see about it. I recalled myself immediately rushing her to the doctor's office without an appointment. I still remember her doctor sighing and saying, "Margaret! Rheumatoid arthritis was enough, and now breast cancer too?"

My mother was treated some thirty years ago with a right radical mastectomy axillary lymph dissection(surgical removal of the breast, chest wall muscles and the lymph nodes under the arm). She also received radiation to the surgical site(at the are of the surgery) and to her ovaries. The operation was quite disfiguring, but she did not succumb to the disease.

I arrived at Dr. JR's office within fifteen minutes. I opened the door and there stood Dr. JR greeting me at the door. We went to an examination room. I presented the mammography films to him. He put them on the viewer, scrutinized and examined them noting the two lesions(masses) deep and close to the chest wall on the films of the left breast. He examined both breasts and commented that the lesions on the left breast were difficult to feel or palpate on clinical examination, that both breasts dense on the mammogram films and both are considerably modular by palpation (touching on examination). Dr. JR kept the films and stated that he will have them returned to Dr. Claudia's office after my surgery.

He asked whether or not I intended to have reconstruction (plastic surgery to have a new breast constructed if I needed my breast removed). I told him that that was why I came to him instead of a general surgeon. I intended to have reconstruction and to be made whole. Dr. JR called the medical center surgery department and scheduled me for an open biopsy for the next morning. Dr. JR later took before-surgery photographs of my breasts which were picture perfect for now, but I knew that that would not be the case 24 hours from now. I thanked him and got dressed and told him that I would see him in the morning.

I got into my Beamer and scurried back to my office. I made arrangements with another physician for coverage of my practice for Friday. I called the hospital administrator and informed him that I would be having a biopsy the next morning. I was almost ready to perform the afternoon surgical tissue examinations, but first I called a short meeting with the laboratory staff. I had learned years ago, about the rumor mill in this town, especially when it concerns physicians' health matters. Rumors spread quite rapidly in the medical community and I wanted my staff to hear about my medical condition directly from me.

I told them that I just had a mammogram that looked highly suspicious for breast cancer. Some of the technicians were teary-eyed by my announcement. I told them that Dr. JR had scheduled my surgical biopsy for tomorrow morning across town. I informed them that the results of the biopsy would more than likely be positive. I let them know that I would be back to work on Monday morning. I told them that I knew their prayers were with me and that I didn't think that the diagnosis would effect my practice and that I was not going to die of the disease, after all I had a mother who lived 26 years after she was diagnosed and treated for her breast cancer and she did not succumb to the disease.

I left the office early and arrived home early for once, by 4:30 p.m.

I still had to break the news to a close friend, who at that time had been recently devastated by the death of his younger brother who had been diagnosed with pancreatic cancer. I told him and he stared and asked, "Why is this happening?" I profoundly told him that just maybe it was happening so that he could be shown how to proceed later in life if he ever received a cancer diagnosis. I told him that there is a lot to cope with when hearing the word cancer from your physician.

Lessons To Be Learned

1) If you feel a mass on breast self examination (BSE) use a marker to put an mark on the area where you feel the mass so that your physician can know where you felt that mass.
2) If your physician does not feel the mass you felt, make sure that you are seen again or if you are at high risk ask for a mammogram.
3) If you have a family history of first degree relatives (a mother or sister) with breast cancer, you are at high risk for the disease. Have your physician give you a risk assessment for breast cancer.
4) Physician recommendations that you should start to have a mammograms at age 35 or age 40 or at age 50 are recommendations only. You should be followed more closely is you are at higher risk for the disease.
5) When you go in for your gynecology exam and your pap smear, make sure that your breasts are examined too. It should be part of the physical exam as well.

THE BIOPSY

I arrived across town at the medical center at 5:30 AM, bright-eyed and bushy tailed. There had been some changes in the outpatient surgery department since my residency in pathology. The head of each patient's bed had been rotated 180 degrees so that the nursing staff could readily see each patient's face in order to monitor their status after the pre-op medication was given. The reason for this change was because there had been an incident a few months prior. A young male patient who received Valium as pre-op medication, had a respiratory arrest, he had stopped breathing and died before he was ever taken to surgery.

I was given the pre-op without incident. Dr. JR came to my bedside and I was wheeled into the surgical suite for the procedure. He reiterated what surgery he was performing on me today, an open biopsy with frozen section (sampling or removal of a portion of the tumor for immediate diagnosis in which a portion of the tissue removed is frozen and slides of the tissue are made for examination by the pathologist under the microscope). I agreed that I understood what procedure was being performed and on what site. He them left and said that he would later see me in surgery.

When I reached the operating suite, I heard the sound of pop music. I was wheeled into the surgery suite. The room was frigid. Why is it always so cold in the surgical suite? I was offered a warm blanket. I welcomed the warm blanket provided by the surgical nursing staff. It reminded of when I would fall asleep on the couch as a child and later become aware of my mother lovingly covering me with a warm blanket.

I was told by the anesthetist to count backwards from ten. I started to count and the next thing I remembered was being in a hospital room when I awoke. Dr. JR came to my room and said that a frozen section, or quick section (tissue removed from the tumor which frozen and immediately examined by the pathologist in the laboratory for evaluation and diagnosis) was performed and that the result was malignant or cancer for both biopsies of the tumor masses. He stated that he would schedule the mastectomy for the next week. I told him that he should schedule it for Friday, because I did not want to miss too much work. He assented.

I was driven home for the day. When arrived home I got

undressed. I looked at the bandages on my left breast, knowing full well that my breast is here today but that this time next week, it would be gone. I couldn't cry. I just wanted to live. I did not want to die. I had no pain. I went to the bathroom to disrobe. I took off my bra and I looked at my left breast with the bandage in place, the evidence that I had had a procedure. They are now no longer the same, I thought. They will never be the same again. I rested over the weekend and reflected on the next step.

I went back to work on Monday morning. I later arranged for coverage of my Pathology Department practice with another pathology group for next Friday, the day of my surgery. I received the biopsy report results later that morning. The diagnosis was ductal carcinoma in situ, comedo-type (cancer involving the breast ducts(tubules or glands, and confined to the ducts. See **Fig. 18.23**.) The biopsy did not show evidence of spread of the tumor outside the ducts. The cancer or tumor cells were confined to the ducts.

That evening I spoke with my Dad, my two brothers and my four sisters and told them about my condition. I told my sisters that they needed to get their mammograms earlier than the current recommended guidelines and that this disease may occur earlier in our generation than it did in our mother. I also urged them to be vigilant with monthly breast self-examinations, even though I didn't think that it did much for me. Within less than a week all of my sisters scheduled mammograms, including the youngest who was twenty-three years old. My sister Karen had a breast mass on mammography. She later had surgery to have the mass removed. The mass was proved to be a benign (non-cancerous) mass or fibroadenoma.

Lessons To Be Learned

1) Before you go to surgery make sure that you know why you are having the surgery, what type of procedure you are having, how it is done and what the complications you may experience by having the procedure. (This is usually discussed in with you in surgeon's office. If you have any questions at that time you should ask them. If you have problems understanding be sure to take someone with you who can ask questions and help you understand. Prior to or on the day of surgery the procedure will again be discussed and you will be asked to sign a permit for surgery which will list the procedure, its indications, possible complications and what has been discussed you.

2) Be sure to ask you doctor for any instructions that he/she may have for you on the day of surgery.

MY TREATMENT AND RECOVERY

It was Friday morning, the day of the scheduled mastectomy(surgical removal of the breast), the day I would lose my left breast and the one part of my body that I was most proud about. My breasts were just the right size. How would I feel after I loss part of my femaleness and my fundamental nature. You may wonder why, so drastic a treatment, why not a lumpectomy (removal of the breast mass and not the entire breast). My left breast had multicentric (multiple-site) disease, two masses in the same breast, not one and the medical thought at that time was that we are dealing with a breast with multifocal disease or breast cancer involving multiple sites and a simple mastectomy with axillary node dissection would be the most appropriate treatment. However, now if a breast had two masses, a lumpectomy of both masses would be an option for treatment.

I checked in the hospital at 5:30 a.m. About a half hour later, was wheeled to the surgery department. Dr. JR came to my bedside and said, "You know that I have scheduled the mastectomy of the left breast with removal of the axillary lymph nodes(lymphn nodes under the arm)? This is the only surgery that I intend to do." I answered, "Yes". He later stated, "You know that the tumor masses are close to the chest wall muscles?". I again stated, "Yes." He stated, "If the muscle is involved, I will take the muscle?" I answered, "Yes, I know."

During the surgical procedure frozen sections (quick sections of tissue to be frozen) near the chest muscle were taken and immediately sent to the pathology lab for analysis. The pathologist's results were immediately reported to Dr. JR. The good news was that the chest wall muscle was not involved. Dr. JR proceeded with the left simple mastectomy and axillary lymph node dissection (removal of the left breast with removal of the lymph nodes under the left arm).

I stayed in the hospital overnight. The next morning Dr. JR came to my bedside with a surgical resident and said that it was okay for me to be dismissed. The resident who came with him asked why I was being dismissed so early. Dr. JR told him that he knew that I would be able to take care of myself and that there was no reason to keep me especially since he knew that I didn't want to be in the hospital. He knew as I did that the sooner that I got back to work the better off I would be.

I was visited a few minutes later by Dr. C. an oncologist (a physician who treats cancer with drugs, chemotherapy) and a fellow medical school classmate of mine. The pathology report was discussed. Both tumor masses were ductal carcinoma in situ; comedo type (see **Figure 18-23**) and one of the tumors had minimal stromal invasion or a small focus of tumor cells that were invading the tissue outside the breast duct. Twenty-six axillary lymph nodes (lymph nodes under the arm) were recovered and all were negative for malignancy(cancer). I asked Dr. C. what his recommendation for further treatment was.

At that time there were two oncological studies, one at Mayo Clinic, and the other at M.D. Anderson. If I had been a patient at Mayo, I would have been offered chemotherapy. If I were a patient in M.D. Anderson no further treatment would be offered. Dr. C. was willing to go along with either decision. I told Dr. C. that I felt that chemotherapy was not needed at this time since there was no documented spread of the tumor into lymphatics and no lymph node involvement. I also told him that my mother had been a breast cancer survivor and she lived some twenty-six years after her diagnosis and did not succumb to the disease. I felt that the course of my disease would be similar.

Dr. C also discussed the fact my cancer had positive estrogen and progesterone receptors (tumor hormone receptors). I had been currently taking the estrogen supplement, Premarin .625 mg daily for a surgically induced menopause, removal of my uterus, fallopian tubes and ovaries, 2 years previously. I told Dr. C. at that time that I would cease taking the hormone since my tumor receptors were positive and since oral estrogen (Premarin) theoretically would promote growth of the tumor.

I was dismissed from the hospital early in the afternoon. I had no significant pain. The first thing on my agenda was to look normal and to be restored so I drove directly to Reiger's Medical Supply Store to be fitted for a breast prosthesis. It is worthy to note that although most women wear bras and think that they know their bra size, very few are properly fitted for a bra. So in essence, many women are wearing an incorrect bra size. A proper fit is necessary for posture and support.

If your bra is uncomfortable or squeezes or flattens you or if you have flab hanging over your bra, then you are not wearing the proper size cup. Even before my surgery I had always hated wearing a bra. I would go free most of the time; my breasts were firm enough and so far had defied gravity, so I didn't really feel the need one. Whenever I wore a bra I could never get it off my mind that I was wearing one. It was quite irritating to me. The only thing that I could think about was getting back home to take it off. I had always thought that my bra cup size was 34 B, but during my fitting I found out that I was actually a 34 C. No wonder why I hated wearing a bra. The properly fitted bra did not squeeze me or pinch my skin. I had no skin bulges and it was made out of a soft comfortable cotton.

There were several prostheses available to choose from. Many of the prostheses were foam and not weighted. I preferred the weighted silicone prosthesis Anemone. This prosthesis felt similar to the normal breast by touch and was of a similar mass and weight. This is extremely important for symmetry. It fit easily into the insert of the post mastectomy surgical bra.

Even though I wore the weighted prosthesis, I was acutely aware that I had a tendency to favor and protect my left side. I stopped using my seat belt in my car while I was driving, because I didn't want anything touching my chest. I also had to make a conscious effort not to slump to the left side.

On the second day after my surgery, the dreaded HOT FLASHES began. I didn't think that I could cope with it very long. During the day, I started flashing and my scalp and face are dripping with sweat. I would awake in the middle of the night with my nightgown was soaked from perspiration. Is this what my mother went through when she received radiation to her ovaries? How did she put up with this? She never complained. I used to she her sweat, but I thought nothing of it. I knew that I would put up with this for as long as I can, but I didn't think that I could keep off of Premarin forever.

I arrived at Dr. JR's office a week later at 9:00 AM. I was scheduled for a post-operative check-up. He said that the surgical site was healing well. He removed my stitches. I was elated that the scar appeared well healed, but I knew from previous surgeries that my well-healed scars usually would break down in the center a few days later after they appeared to be well healed. I was hoping that this would not be the case this time.

Dr. JR took more photographs. He said that I would be able to start reconstruction in January. I told him that I was thinking that around Thanksgiving time would be best since the surgical site would be well healed by that time. He stated that the reason he suggested January was because it gives the patient time to get used to the fact that she has no breast and that when she undergoes the reconstruction she is more able to accept and appreciate the reconstructed breast, which will never be the same as the breast that was lost. Dr. JR and I agreed that reconstruction would take place prior to Thanksgiving.

Three days after my post-surgical checkup my wound broke down in its center. I went to Dr. JR's office. There was no infection. The wound will heal by secondary intention meaning that the wound would remain open and the tissue defect would slowly be filled in and be replaced by dense fibrous or scar tissue and the surface skin or epithelium would grow over the scar tissue. The wound healed slowly and left a hypertrophic (big thick) scar.

Thanksgiving Reconstruction

I arrived at the hospital for reconstruction at 6:00 A.M. I was going to receive a submuscular(beneath the muscle) Dow Corning silicone implant. A pocket was formed beneath the pectoralis chest muscle, which had been partially freed from the chest wall. The implant was inserted in the pocket beneath my pectoralis chest muscle and a drainage device was placed laterally. When I left the operating suite and awaked in post-op care, I was in no pain. I was then transferred to the floor. My pain medication was no longer effective by the time I reached my room. I summoned the nurse. She gave me Talwin for pain and it only made me vomit.

It did not help that I also had the roommate from "Hell" who just had an endometrial scraping (a sampling of the tissue lining the uterus cavity removed) performed. She was talking incessantly on the telephone and full of jabber. Her surgery was in no way comparable to mine. The pain of a few minor uterine cramps can in no way compare with the amount of pain that I was experiencing. Just imagine someone taking a clamp and pulling the muscles off of your chest. The pain was excruciating and unrelenting. I knew that I had to get out of that hospital bed as soon as possible and go home or else the nurses would have a difficult and combative patient on their hands my roommate did not stop talking.

I called the nurse and told her that I was ready to go home. She brought me a prescription for Talwin and told me that I was to follow-up with the doctor on next Thursday. She told me that I was not to return to work until after my visit with the doctor in a week. I said okay and wished her a Happy Thanksgiving. By 11:15 A.M., I was on the elevator and by 11:30A.M. I was being driven home.

The pain continued. I did not take any Talwin or Tylenol #3 because I did not like how I felt after taking pain medications. I was resolved to block the pain out in my mind. I went to sleep. When I awoke the pain had diminished. I slept for a few hours more.

I was truly thankful when Thanksgiving Day came. I was thankful that I did not have to wear the prosthesis anymore. I looked at myself in the mirror. I now had a mound or a simulated breast. My surgical scar will not show when I wear a low cut evening or cocktail dress because Dr. JR made a horizontal surgical incision.

By Monday morning, my pain was suppressed and I felt that I could return to work, so I did so against my Doctor's advice. Thursday morning, I went in for my post-op checkup. When I went into the office, Dr. JR was grinning ear-to-ear and asked, "Well, how do you feel? I didn't tell you how much pain you would have after that surgery!" I told him that I was in intense pain after the surgery and that I did not take any pain medications since the first Talwin that a received before I left the hospital. I told him that I blocked the pain out with my mind and that I felt fine. I also told him that I had started back to work on Monday. He shook his head, he just couldn't believe that I was in no pain and that I was able to block out the pain. I told him that some people are capable of doing this and can set their pain thresholds higher when necessary. Now when I reflect about it, it was most likely by the grace of God that the pain diminished so swiftly.

Dr. JR took post-surgical photographs and discussed the next surgical procedure, the construction of a new areola or nipple. Dr. JR stated that he did not know what part of the body that the skin should come from. He stated that on Caucasians the skin is usually obtained from the upper inner thigh, which is more hyperpigmented. I told him that for Black people the skin of the upper inner thigh is also hyperpigmented and that that is where the skin should be taken. He was surprised. I told him that there are different races of people but we are all pretty much anatomically the same. The surgery was scheduled for mid-May.

Christmas was coming and I decided that this was going to have my best Christmas ever, since I did not know if I would ever see another one again. I put up a Christmas tree in every room of the house. Evergreen garlands draped the staircase, both fireplaces and the balcony rails of the great room. I had a party with some thirty guests. I was quite the hostess. I had the meal catered. Everyone enjoyed themselves. The old year left and the New Year came in with a big bang.

Areola (Nipple) Reconstruction

Winter faded and spring came in anew. I spent some time planting flowers. When I saw Dr. JR in May at the medical center before the procedure I had one request. He asked what was the request. I asked him to please put the areolar skin at the same level as the other breast. He asked why I requested this and I told him because when my clothes were off, I wanted the nipples to be at the same level when I stand in front of the mirror, since the normal breast sags a little when compared with the new mound.

When I awoke from the procedure a 4x2 cm strip of skin had been removed from my right upper inner thigh. Thick suture (surgical thread) had been used to close the wound. The sutures had been pulled tight. A circular portion of skin had been removed from the mound and the newly excised skin from the thigh was used for areola or nipple construction. It was centrally placed at that site. The nipple was protected by as small plastic cylindrical device.

Before I left the hospital a beautiful tropical floral arrangement containing Birds of Paradise flowers arrived. The card accompanying arrangement stated, "Congratulations on your new baby!" It was from the hospital interns. They later told me that they wanted to send me flowers and they didn't know what to say, but thought that the card they sent was
and they didn't know what to say, but thought that the card they sent was

and they didn't know what to say, but thought that the card they sent was completely appropriate and said it all. What a great class!

Postoperatively, I had no significant pain in the area of reconstruction. I removed my sutures within a week. Dr. JR said that he wanted the sutures in the upper inner thigh to remain for two weeks. By the end of week one, my skin became somewhat inflamed, but I was determined to keep the sutures in for the full two weeks. By the end of the next week both upper inner thighs were inflamed and the skin moist, weeping and sensitive. I called Dr. JR and asked him if I could remove the sutures, because both legs were now equally swollen and irritated. He assented. I removed sutures. After removing the sutures I felt much, much better. The inflammatory reaction resolved within four days.

The month of June soon came. My intern class was graduating. I attended the yearly intern graduating ceremonies. I felt whole. I was able to wear a black short evening dress with a low neckline. Many present atthe reception would never know the ordeal that I had been through in the past year just by looking at me. This entire process of being whole had been important to me and the ordeal was well worth it.

My aunt who had had a mastectomy in the 1950s said that it was just not that important. I told her that it was important to me since I was single. She assured me that a mastectomy was not important to men. Just maybe she was right. I was told this by my friend, "Woman, I would love you and will love you if you have two breasts, one breast or no breasts at all. Ah, I just love the woman!"

Even after all the surgeries, it was brought up to me that I was still favoring and protecting the left side of my chest. I still tended to walk with my left shoulder slightly lower than the right. I was still protective of the left side of my chest and still not wearing a car seat belt. I resolved that I would now make a concerted effort to correct my posturing.

Staying Healthy Alive and Well!

One of the last things that my Mother said to me about a month before she died was, "Continue exercising. It is very important that you do so!" This comment seemed very strange to me at the time, especially since athletics had not been stressed to me by my parents as having any importance in life. Education was stressed and considered extremely important to my parents. They made sure that we attended private Catholic and elementary school and high school. My Dad had always said, "Gym class doesn't matter!"

Maybe my mother could see herself in me and knew that it would be extremely important for my survival to maintain a healthy weight. My mother had been prescribed the steroid, Prednisone(an anti-inflammatory or drug that suppresses the body's immune system) for her rheumatoid arthritis when she was young and suffered from the long term effects of being on steroids. I had been prescribed the steroid, Prednisone and Benadryl, (an anti-histamine) for an allergic or immune skin disorder. My cholesterol was high and I was about twenty pounds over my ideal weight. I asked my dermatologist what did she recommended for her patients with high cholesterol levels because of the steroids and receive no answer from her. She stated that no patient had ever asked her that before.

I was thirty-four years old now and I knew that what condition I was in now and how I continued would affect the remainder of my life. One of my professors from medical school used to ask us as students, What do you want to do when you grow up? The question for me now is, how do you want to live and what changes are you going to make to stay healthy for the rest of your life? What quality of life do you want to have for the rest of your life? I had made a decision to continue taking my daily Premarin, an estrogen replacement hormone. At that time there were not any other suitable medical alternatives for treatment. This was probably not the decision I should make, but the hot flashes had been intolerable for me. My sleeping patterns were disturbed by the hot flashes at night. My hair was matted each morning because it became soaking wet during the night. I just couldn't take it any longer. I knew that there was a risk for breast cancer recurrence because of the use of exogenous estrogens, but I also knew that my mother lived some twenty-six years after the diagnosis of her breast cancer with no recurrence. There are other cells in my body at my young age that needed estrogen.

I joined a hard-core free weight gym that had members who were competitive body builders, who were constantly preparing for competitive meets. I became very muscular and lost weight. I discovered that I was an extremely good athlete and that there had always been a little athlete inside if me that had been crying to be free.

Six months later, I joined a girly gym with aerobics training, Olympic swimming pool, sauna, steam room and a free-weight room because I did not want to have a bulky look. I just wanted to be fit and lose the majority of my body fat to decrease the possibility of a reoccurrence of the breast cancer. Vigorous exercise would also combat the catabolic (breakdown) effects of the steroid, prednisone on the body. I had been taking because of my skin condition. I needed to reverse the water retention, the high cholesterol levels and the risk of osteoporosis (bone loss). I started taking over the counter Niacin (Vitamin B3), 1,000 mg daily to reduce the high cholesterol levels. My high density lipoprotein (HDL) levels were already high and protective for my heart status.

The exercise was paying off. I was able to reduce the amount of steroids I was taking. I went from a size 10 dress size to a size 6. My diet changed in that I was eating more fresh fruits and vegetables. I was also eating more often. When a person is physically fit the body tends to dictate what it needs. You are more in tune with your physical needs. There is no mental imperative for binge eating.

I continued my yearly mammograms, but within a few years those exams became 1 year and three months to every other year or when my physician's office called me requesting that it be done. It is good to have a physician that makes sure that you keep up with your examinations as recommended.

I became an advocate in the fight against breast cancer. I was the Chair of the American Cancer Society's Breast Cancer Task Force, in my area with members from all local breast cancer support organizations, areas hospitals, radiology departments, clinics and advocate breast cancer survivors. The task force goals were to determine the hindrances to access of mammography screening and programs in rural parts of the state, to advocate mammography screening, monthly breast self examinations and yearly examinations by a physician. The task force was also interested in the increased mastectomy rates as the primary treatment for breast cancer in my state at that time when compared to the national level. Through our efforts a state law was passed making it mandatory that all women receive the information that they needed on choices of surgical treatment, i.e. simple mastectomy with or without axillary node dissection and/or lumpectomy (surgical removal of breast mass or lump) with axillary lymph nodes sampling (sampling of lymph nodes under the arm). During my time as serving as chair at least three survivor members of the Task Force succumbed to this dreaded disease, one was the facilitator of the task force. She was young, only 32 years old, full of life, married with two children and had been diagnosed with breast cancer at the age of 28 years. I can only admire such women who untiringly give of themselves to help others and impart hope even when they are struggling for their own lives.

Lesson To Be Learned

1) Before you go to surgery make sure that you know why you are having the surgery, what type of procedure you are having, how it is done and what the complications you may experience by having the procedure. (This is usually discussed in with you in surgeon's office. If you have any questions at that time you should ask them. If you have problems understanding be sure to take someone with you who can ask questions and help you understand. Prior to or on the day of surgery the procedure will again be discussed and you will be asked to sign a permit for surgery which will list the procedure, its indications, possible complications and what has been discussed you.

2) Be sure that your surgeon has discussed the types of surgical procedures for the treatment of breast cancer, i.e. lumpectomy, simple mastectomy, radical mastectomy, axillary lymph node sampling, sentinel node biopsy (the first node draining the cancer) and axillary lymph node dissection.

3) If you are considering breast reconstruction, consider you options for the types of reconstruction available and discuss them with your surgeon and consider when reconstruction would be better for you and what type of procedure would be best for you based upon the timing of other treatments which you may undergo based on the extent of your disease.

4) Be sure to ask you doctor for any instructions that he/she may have for you on the day of surgery.

5) After treatment, get on a good exercise program and eat a diet low in fat with fresh fruit, vegetables and fiber (See Chapter 30).

THE SECOND TIME AROUND

THE RIGHT UNDERARM MASS

It was February 2001, mid-winter, when I noticed a reddened pea sized area of the skin of my left breast in the lower outer quadrant. The area was suggestive of a bug bite. There was no scaling of the skin. There was no firmness of the breast tissue noted. The redness disappeared in a few days.

In March I noted a rubbery freely movable, not hardened, non-painful nodule under my right arm. I thought that it might be a benign (non-cancerous) fat nodule or lipoma. I had my husband feel it. I had never had a case of hidradenitis (abscess or inflammation involving sweat ducts in the underarm area), although my Mother was plagued with such during her teens. The area was not gross inflammation, or redness and hotness of the area to touch. There were no skin changes. There was no pain. My husband applied a hot compress to the area and within the next three days, the nodule or mass disappeared.

I had planted a one-half bushel of yellow and white daffodils bulbs in the fall and I and was now seeing the fruits of my labor as winter was ushered out and spring emerged. The daffodils were beginning to sprout. I spent a lot of time in the following weeks after work, clearing the flowerbeds from dead leaves and dried plants. I planted variegated orange and yellow marigolds, and white, yellow, pink, lavender and purple pansies, caladiums, and elephant ears. I also planted a few shrubs, forsythias and Roses of Sharon.

By the end of May I noted some soreness in my right upper arm. My husband told me that I had been doing too much yard work. He asked me if I had sprung my shoulder at work by lifting a body during an autopsy. I told him not to my knowledge. Over the summer the pain did not resolve and it became worse and unrelenting. I took no analgesics or pain medicines. My sister who was living overseas was coming home for the summer. I was looking forward to making the shopping trips that she and my other sister would be making.

We started shopping in July. We hit the malls on the east and west side of town, shopping areas in the burbs, small towns within thirty mile radius from the city and of course Target and Wal-Mart. We shopped until I dropped literally. My sisters had to help me with some of my packages and bags because my right arm was hurting. By the end of August, I decided to investigate what I had been procrastinating about and hoping that it wasn't so.

During the last three months as pathologist, I had examined multiple surgical specimens, which presented as masses under the arm. The diagnoses varied from lymphadenitis suppurativa (abscesses involving lymph nodes in the axilla), metastatic breast cancer (breast cancer which had spread to the lymph nodes under the arm), metastatic melanoma (malignant melanoma skin cancer which had spread to the lymph nodes under the arm), cat scratch disease (disease caused by a cat scratch which causes inflammation and abscesses of the lymph nodes under the arm), and malignant lymphoma (a malignancy originating from the cells within the lymph nodes). I vowed that my procrastination was over. There was now a mass under my arm which was hard, fixed and non-movable. I picked up the telephone and called my surgeon friend Dr. JP. I told him that I thought that I had a mass in the right axilla (in the right underarm area). He told me that he was in the hospital on the surgical floor. He said that he would be right down.

Dr. J.P. came straight to my office. I closed the mini-blinds in my office and let him examine me. He confirmed the presence of the mass. We planned to set the surgery for next Tuesday. I came home and told my husband. He did not want me to have surgery at all and definitely not on that day. I told him that I needed to have the surgery. He reluctantly agreed to my rescheduling the surgery for the next week late Friday afternoon, that way it would not interfere with my work schedule and I could recuperate over the weekend.

Lessons To Be learned

1) Never procrastinate, never put off, never delay. If you notice something wrong, a reddened area or rash on the skin of the breast, a breast lump or mass or a lymph under the arm or in the neck, see your physician. Procrastination results in a delay in diagnosis.
2) Any pain in the shoulder area or under the arm is significant. It could be a warning sign of breast cancer.

SURGERY AGAIN

I arrived at the surgery suite after I had examined the last surgical specimen of the day. My husband was present. Dr. JP spoke with him. I had a local anesthetic. The mass that was removed was placed on the surgical dumb-waiter and sent to pathology. Within an hour after the procedure, I put on my clothes and went to the lab. The histotechnologist was still there waiting for me to process the specimen. My husband accompanied me to the laboratory. He watched as I showed him the firm yellow tan mass with areas which were softened or necrotic. The mass was up to 3 by 2 cm. I made sections through it with a sharp surgical knife and made two dab or imprint smears on a glass slide by lightly touching two glass slides with the tissues cut surfaces in multiple areas of the mass. Representative sections from the tumor mass were submitted for routine tissue processing and placed in small rectangular cassettes which would later be placed in the tissue processor. The imprint or dab smears on the slides were immediately placed in alcohol and later the slides were stained by the histotechnologist.

My husband and I went to my office. The histotechnologist brought the stained slides to me so that I could evaluate them under the microscope and make a diagnosis. My husband looked on the other side of my dual-head microscope. I examined the first slide and said to my husband, "It is metastatic breast cancer." I could only imagine what he may have been thinking or what he was imagining at that time. I prepared part of the specimen to be sent to a referral laboratory for other studies, estrogen and progesterone hormonal steroid receptors, HER2 (test for a biomarker or gene associated with an aggressive form of breast cancer) and DNA analysis, the analysis of cancer cells synthesizing DNA. My husband and I went home and I recuperated over the weekend.

Lessons To Be Learned

1) Breast cancer is evaluated by the pathologist. The pathologist examines, cuts and looks at prepared slides to evaluate the tumor. Besides the evaluation under the microscope, certain tests may also be done to further classify the tumor. This includes ER and

PR (estrogen and progesterone) steroid hormone receptors, the HER2 biomarker and DNA analysis of the cancer cells.

PATHOLOGY REPORT, EXAMINATION AND STAGING

On Monday morning, I read the routine surgical pathology cases for the day and my tissue slides. The tumor diagnosis was a poorly differentiated infiltrating ductal carcinoma (an invasive duct, tubule or gland cancer with poor tubule development). There was replacement of the lymph node by cancer cells. I sent via the laboratory courier, a copy of my surgical pathology report to Dr. E., my colleague and an oncologist. I received a phone call from Dr. E. the next morning. He stated that he received a pathology report with my name typed on it as the patient and asked if it was my report. I told him yes. He said that he would be coming to the lab later that morning.

Dr. E later came to my office. He told me to get the following tests done: Chemistry panel with liver profile(tests for liver function), complete blood count (count of red and white cells in the blood and platelets), serum CA-125 (cancer tumor marker in the blood for ovarian cancer), CEA (cancer tumor marker in the blood for adenocarcinoma or duct and gland cancers), a bone scan, liver scan, CT scan thorax and abdomen and a MUGA heart scan, a test is used to make precise measurements of cardiac pumping function. This test is most often used to monitor the effects of chemotherapy that can potentially damage the heart. I told him that I would have the tests done. I later had my blood drawn by one of the phlebotomists in the lab and called outpatient scheduling to set up the radiological exams.

The next afternoon I had a CT scan, a bone scan and liver scan. There were no abnormalities of the liver and bone scan. There was an abnormality noted by CT scan. There was an 8 millimeter subcutaneous (under the skin) nodule in the left lower quadrant of the left breast. As I am sure you remember it was sixteen years previously that I had had a left mastectomy with axillary node dissection and later reconstruction of the left breast with a submuscular implant. The radiologist requested diagnostic bilateral mammograms.

The next morning as soon as there was a lag in my schedule in the laboratory I went to radiology for the diagnostic mammograms. My breasts were quite tender that day, especially the upper outer quadrant of my right breast, which was near the recent surgical site. The radiologic technician completed the examination of the right breast and axilla. Multiple studies were performed on the left breast and implant. Markers were placed on the previous old surgical scar. Since there was minimal skin and soft tissue present, manipulation of the left breast was quite painful. I shouted, "Enough is enough! I can't take it no more!" I went back to my office.

About an hour later Dr. GW, a radiation oncologist belonging to the same group as Dr. E. came to my office. He was there to console me. I told him that I was upset and that I couldn't finish the mammography study of my left breast and that I was tired of my sore boobs being squashed multiple times just because a male radiologist wants to get the perfect picture of the density in my left breast, especially since there is hardly no tissue there to begin with. I also told him that at this moment I did not want another person to touch me or order any more tests on me, especially a flat chested male who doesn't even have breasts. Dr. GW. said, "If you don't want a male radiologist, you don't have to have a male radiologist. I'll call my friend across town and she can complete the studies." I assented.

The next day I went across town to a female radiologist, Dr. B. I gave her copies of the previous studies that had been completed and went for a more extensive examination. Yes, it hurt just as much as the films that were ordered by the male radiologist, but at least this time a female ordered the studies and she had been through the procedure multiple times herself and had had surgical biopsies of her breasts. It may seem silly but at that moment, I just wanted someone that had previously been put through the drill, someone who could be empathetic and as gentle as possible.

The study confirmed the presence of the nodule in the left lower quadrant of the left breast as noted by the CT scan. There was also a suspicious area in the right upper quadrant of the right breast. Dr. B said that she could do an ultrasound of both breasts today, now at 4:00 PM, for my convenience and perform needle biopsies of both lesions. I said okay and we walked over to the main hospital.

The ultrasound room was slightly larger than most radiology rooms. A technician was present and a nurse to administer a medication for pain. I told Dr. B that it would be unnecessary and that I would not be in any pain. The nurse stayed anyway, just in case. The skin of the breast was prepped (cleaned and sterilized) in the lower outer quadrant of the left breast first. The ultrasound technician localized the left breast lesion, which was less than 1 cm in size. Dr. B used an automatic needle biopsy to obtain the core biopsies. She asked me whether or not I was in pain after the first biopsy. I told her that I felt only a scraping gritty movement and that there was no pain. She obtained three more needle cores biopsies (cylindrical cores of tissue), which were placed in a small bottle containing the clear formalin fixative.

Dr. B then prepped the skin of the upper outer quadrant of the right breast. The ultrasound technician localized the area that was in question. It was not as discrete as the lesion in the left breast. Dr. B was seeing a density that was somewhat irregular with a central blood vessel. She knew of my clinical history of hypersensitivity vasculitis (an inflammatory condition of blood vessels) and asked me what it would look like under the microscope. I told her that it would be a blood vessel with a cuff or collar of lymphocytes (a type of white blood cells or inflammatory cells) surrounding it. She said, "This is probably what this density is. It looks like a blood vessel with a white cuff around it." She took four core biopsies from the area and placed them in another labeled container with formalin fixative.

Dr. B then placed bandages over both biopsy areas. I was given ice packs and told to keep them in place to lessen swelling and bruising. I placed both ice packs in my bra. While I was putting on my blouse, Dr. B called the pathology department and spoke to Dr. R. who told her that someone was available in the department to receive the specimen and make sure that it was processed so that it could be examined the next day. I thanked Dr. B and told her that I would be in touch. I left the medical facility and returned to my office across town to close it for the day.

I later drove home. When I arrived my husband asked, "What happened to you?" I told him that I was okay and that I had just had needle core biopsies of both breasts and that the ice packs were to stay in place until the ice melted. I told him that I had had diagnostic mammograms performed across town and that ultrasounds were also done. Instead of having to make another appointment for the needle core biopsies I had them done at that time, that way I would get the results the next day. He had to laugh a little and so did I, because suddenly I looked like I had enormous breasts with the ice packs in place. I left them in place until the ice melted. I had no bleeding nor swelling.

The next morning when I was in the office I received a phone call from Dr. DC, a pathologist and colleague in the pathology department of medical center across town, whom I have known for a long time. He confirmed the biopsies from the left breast as poorly differentiated infiltrating ductal carcinoma. He wanted to know if I needed estrogen and progesterone receptors and Her2Neu. I told him that I have the results of a biopsy from a mass from the right axilla and that the further studies would not be needed. He told me that the result of the biopsy from the right breast was benign perivasculitis with fat necrosis (inflammation, inflammatory cells around a blood vessel with necrosis or degeneration of the fat). I told him that it correlates with the results of the ultrasound. I thanked him for calling me and he wished me good luck.

Dr. EE, my oncologist later stopped by my office. He said the results of the MUGA heart scan was normal and that I should be able to take the chemotherapy drug, Adriamycin. He also stated that he wanted Dr. JP to completely remove any residual axillary lymph nodes and to remove the nodule in the left breast. I told Dr. JP of Dr EE's recommendations. Dr. JP was worried that I might get a paraesthesia (weakness and numbness of the larm) since the dissection planes of the tissue under the right arm may not be distinct because of the previous surgical procedure. I informed Dr. EE of this. Dr. JP said that he would try. Surgery was scheduled for late next Friday.

I arrived to the surgery department ready for my procedure. Dr. EE told me to tell Dr. JP that if he was not able to complete the resection that it would be okay. I however, told him that he did not have to worry and that God has helped and that he would find that the anatomical planes were still intact so that he could complete the resection. He asked me if I needed to go to x-ray first to have the nodule or tumor in the left breast localized so that he could resect it. I told him that it wasn't necessary and told him where the lesion was by pointing to it. I told him that it was very small and could be removed with an ellipse of skin. I pointed to it, but he couldn't feel it. He told the nurse place an "X" on the spot as I so designated.

When I awoke from the surgery, my husband was at my bedside. I was glad he came. I do so know how much he hates hospitals and their medicinal smell. I stopped in the lab and saw my specimens. My histotechnologist was still there. She had numbered the tissue cassettes so that I could submit representative sections of the specimens for examination under the microscope.

I performed a gross examination of the lumpectomy specimen from the left breast. It consisted of an elliptical wedge of skin and soft tissue. There was no gross tumor on the margins of excision. The tumor on cut section was up to 8 mm across. The margins were inked with a black surgical pathology marker and I submitted sections and placed them into the small rectangular cassettes for tissue processing. The right axillary or underarm contents consisted of up to seven lymph nodes within adipose tissue or fat. No gross tumor was noted in the lymph nodes. The lymph nodes were submitted into cassettes. The tissue was to be processed over the weekend and the slides would be examined under the microscope on Monday.

The weekend was uneventful. I had no discomfort. My left and right breasts looked slightly more symmetrical. I went to my office Monday morning and reviewed my slides. There were no surprises. Copies of the report were sent to Drs. EE and JP. The receptionist from Dr. EE's office called to set up an appointment for me to see him. I made the appointment for Thursday afternoon.

I had been having a lot of trouble sleeping lately. I would retire at midnight, awake at 3:00 AM. and would not get back to sleep until 5:00 AM. This was rather disconcerting since I had to get to work by 8:00 AM. I needed my sleep more, especially now.

Lessons To Be Learned

1) The oncologists usually requests other laboratory and radiology tests and scans to assess the extent of the spread of the tumor to lymph nodes, other organs and bone in order to determine the stage of the cancer.
2) Diagnostic mammographys are performed for the assessment of lesions that are detected. Such examinations could influence

treatment decisions in lesions that are small in size.

3) Ultrasound is another modality used to examine the breast and lesions that are detectable on mammography.This examination can help detect the area where the radiologist will obtain the tissue core biopsies.

4) Needle core biopsies are performed to diagnose lesions which may occur on mammography and ultrasound. Small lesions can sometimes be completely removed by this procedure.

5) Sometimes it is necessary to localize a breast lesion with a needle or wire hook with the injections of dyes prior to surgery so that the lesion can be identified and to help the surgeon, so that the correct area can be removed.

THE TREATMENT PLAN

I kept my appointment with Dr. EE on Thursday afternoon. He did a complete physical and discussed treatment options with me. The options would be chemotherapy followed by radiation therapy. He told me that he would schedule for Dr. JP to insert a Port-a-Cath (a device inserted into the subclavian vein with a port placed under the skin of the chest through which chemotherapy drugs are administered into the vein directly). Starting in November I would have four rounds of CA (Cytoxan and Adriamycin) and followed by four rounds of Taxol. Dr. EE told me that since I worked out and carried little body fat, he expected that I would be more toxic than most adults and behave clinically similarly as pediatric (child) patients, since they usually show more toxic symptoms. The chemotherapy treatment would take three months to complete.

I told him that I wanted to be active and work during treatment. He said that it could be possible. He planned to keep my white blood cell counts increased with Neupogen shots and to use Procrit to maintain my red blood cell counts. I told him that I just didn't like the fact that I had to have chemotherapy and in my mind I was still in denial, and somewhat rebellious to the fact that I needed this treatment. I did not want to loose my hair. A Black woman's crowning glory is the length of her hair a very common belief.

I vocalized again to Dr. EE that I didn't want to lose my hair and that it took me so long to grow it to the length that it was. I told him also that I felt that this entire treatment process was too long. He emphatically said that it wasn't and told me that the therapy for leukemias and lymphomas are a lot longer. He emphatically told me that I needed the treatment. My denial and procrastinating stubborn personality was showing. I told him that I had to think about it. I did however make an appointment for Friday the following week for my first day of treatment. I went back to my office and closed shop.

When I drove home I was quite upset. I arrived home and ate some frozen yogurt. Later when my husband came home, I told him that I would probably need chemotherapy. He was not enthused about this statement. I said no more that evening and retired. I awoke again at 3:00AM. I am so, so very tired of this waking up at and not being able to go back to sleep.

I went to work the next morning. I received a phone call from Dr. RR, who is a family practitioner and a close friend of mine. He asked me whether nor not I was going to have chemotherapy. I told him, I didn't want to. He said why not. I told him I didn't want to lose my hair. He said, "You have to have chemotherapy!" He also told me that people don't die just because they have chemotherapy. Most of my patients that have had chemotherapy are alive. I told him that it was good for him to remind me of that fact, because as a pathologist I normally see post-treatment failure biopsies and this does not represent the majority of cases.

Later that afternoon, Dr. EE came to my office. I listened to him. I told him that I still had to decide and reminded him that I just didn't want to lose my hair. I reiterated that to a black woman this hair thing is a vain thing and perceived as a woman's crowning glory. I told him also that I knew that it was going to be a big factor in my discussion at home with my husband, including a discussion on religion, relying on God's healing and discussions on whether or not I pray enough.

When I left the office, I drove around in the parking lot several times. I felt like a chicken that had lost its head. I said to myself, "Stop this! What are you worried about? If you die today where will you be?" I said, "I know, I'll be with God in heaven." From that time forward there was no more worry and no more 3:00 AM awakenings.

I told my husband that I was going to have chemotherapy. Again, he was not enthused. He said that I needed to pray more and then I wouldn't have to have chemotherapy. I told him that I still needed to have chemotherapy. I told him that if he wants me to be around here more than five years then I needed to have chemotherapy. I told him that I wasn't wanting chemotherapy and that I didn't want to lose my hair, but that it was the only thing that would keep me here longer and that I wasn't quite ready to die. I also told him that I had procrastinated and denied that I had cancer too long and that I should have had a biopsy last February when we felt the fullness or lipoma under my arm. I also told him that I had been in pain for the last four months.

I told him that I would be calling my sisters to let them know of my condition and that it was important for me to do so, since there are other options that they may want to consider in their lives so that they don't have to go through what I will be going through.

Later that evening I called my sisters. The one that resided in the same city as I asked me when I was going to have the first treatment. I told her, not this Friday, but on the next Friday afternoon! She said that she would be there. My husband called my Dad and told him that I there was a new treatment that I was going to take to prevent my breast cancer from recurring. We told him this because we did not want him to worry. We also told him that there was nothing risky about the treatment. My father was 82 years old and had had several transient ischemic attacks, TIAs, mini-strokes. We particularly didn't want him to worry especially since we recently loss a 42 year-old cousin with metastatic breast cancer in August less than two months ago. She left an 8 year-old daughter who is now residing with her grandparents.

Lessons To Be Learned

1) Fear, anger, frustration and denial are common reactions when one receives a diagnosis of cancer. Do not let this get in the way of your receiving the treatment that you need to survive and beat breast cancer.

2) Chemotherapy is essential when breast cancer has spread outside the breast and involves lymph nodes. Chemotherapy is necessary to treat the tumor cells Systemically or that may be left in the body and spread into the lymph or blood.

3) Radiation treatments are necessary to treat local disease, near the tumor site.

THE INFAMOUS PORT-A-CATH

Dr. JP inserted the Port-a-Cath on Friday afternoon. It is a dome-shaped metallic device with a rectangular flat base and an elasticized plastic sheath covering the surface into which an intravenous (IV) needle could be inserted to administer the chemotherapy drugs. A piece of white silastic tubing was attached to the device to be pnserted the vein. The Port-a-Cath device itself was placed beneath the skin and the tubing within the subclavian vein.

When I awoke I found my husband at my bedside looking upon me sympathetically and waiting to take me home. I also discovered the 2 cm bulge, sitting on my right chest. I dressed and went home for the weekend. My husband was curious about the device and the bulge on my chest, which was covered by an elastic Band-Aid. I did not take the elastic Band-Aid off, so that he could have a peak though. I told him he would see it soon. He took me home and I immediately undressed, put on my nightgown and went to sleep early. When I awoke in the morning I could barely get out of bed. The Port felt like a heavy weight on my chest. I arose and held on to it because it felt like it was going to fall off my chest. This sensation continued until mid-week, after that I never felt its presence or that sensation again.

THE CHEMOTHERAPY

Round One

The first Friday of November came; I stopped my workday at 2:00 PM and went to my appointment for my chemotherapy treatment. My husband came to my office to accompany me. When I arrived at Dr. EE's office to my surprise not only was my sister there, but also her husband and her two sons. We hugged and greeted each other. My sister, Cynthia said that her sons wanted to come too, because they were worried about me. She asked whether or not it was okay. I replied that I was. I looked around the room and noticed that none of the other patients receiving infusions had loved ones accompanying them. They came by themselves, and were either looking at TV, reading books or newspapers or perusing the pages of a magazine. They all looked at me. An older slightly robust gentleman said, "You must be a newcomer?" I said, "Yes." I didn't have the heart to ask him how he knew. I was the only patient with a whole entourage of people accompanying me.

Dr. EE came out of his back office. He said, "I am so surprised that you are here! You seemed so adamant that you weren't going to take the treatment." I told him, "Denial, denial, denial!" The nurse told me privately that she was so glad that I changed my mind, because she could see that I was not going to make it if I didn't come in for treatment. What a profound statement! If I had wondered where this statement came from, I only had to later look at photographs that were taken of me over the past year to see that I was sick. People should take frequent photographs of their loved ones just to assess the status of their health; subtle changes can be noted over time.

The nurse took my vital signs, temperature and blood pressure. Since I now had bilateral axillary lymph node dissections (removal of lymph nodes under both arms), my right leg was used to obtain my blood pressure to prevent the risk of lymphedema (swelling of the arms due to blocked lymph vessels). The nurse set up the IV (intravenous set up). I was to receive two drugs today, Cytoxan (Cyclophosphamide), and Adriamycin (Doxorubicin).

I wore navy blue wool suite with a lavender sweater, which buttoned in the front in order to provide easy access for the infusions. The nurse removed the bandage from the Port-a-Cath and stated that it would be used to for the infusion of all chemotherapy drugs, and blood draws for all laboratory tests. She asked me if I was allergic to Iodine and I replied no. She then proceeded to clean the surface of the skin covering the port with a Betadine scrub which contained Iodine.

The nurse adjusted the fluid in the IV tubing and said, "I am now going the access the Port. There will be a stick." There was a stick! I felt it! It felt like a ice pick stab as it pierced the skin over the port. Tears rolled down my cheeks for the first time. The nurse asked, "Did I hurt you?" I said crying, "No, it is not that. This is the first time that what I am going through is really affecting me. This is reality. This is really happening to me. I am undergoing chemotherapy and this is really, really happening to me!" My sister Cynthia had tears in her eyes and the nurse also became teary eyed.

It took approximately four hours until the infusion was complete. My sister and my husband stayed until it was completed. I received two injections subcutaneously (in the fat under my skin in the belly), Procrit for red blood cell production and Neupogen for white blood cell production. I ordered additional Neupogen and Procrit from the pharmacy so that I could give the injections to myself daily instead of having to return to the oncology clinic each day. Before the IV was disconnected I also received an IV medication for nausea. I did not want any additional medications for nausea. I felt that I would be able to handle it on my own and tough it out.

The nurse gave me telephone numbers to call if I had any problems. The nurse also told me that I could come to the clinic next Thursday to get my blood drawn for lab tests, a complete blood count and liver profile. There was no way that I was going to come back. I didn't want the Port accessed again. I told her that I would have it drawn at the lab and fax the results.

On the way out my husband asked me how I was feeling. I told him that I felt slightly waterlogged and as is if foreign substances were in my body. I smelled a faint metallic or medicinal odor. I also felt as though my sinuses were being opened up. When we got into the SUV, there was a funny smell. I felt slightly nauseous. After we arrived home, I prepared the dining table for dinner. Before I was finished warming the food, I began to feel more nauseous. My stomach felt hot and I scurried to the bathroom, pushed up the toilet seat and vomited. My husband rushed to help me and soothed my forehead with a cool moist white cotton towel. I thanked him and told him that I was feeling better and could probably eat now. After I ate and washed the dishes, I retired early and called it a day

I slept pretty soundly. When I awakened the next morning, I was famished. I knew that I had to eat now. The chemotherapy drugs are indiscriminate and kill both normal cells and tumor cells. My body was demanding food to make new cells. I ate a hardy breakfast and still felt as if my stomach was a bottomless pit. When I brushed my teeth, I became nauseous. Each time I went into the bathroom I would start to salivate excessively and needed to vomit. My husband just used a dilute solution of bleach to spot clean one of his shirts and I suddenly became nauseous. I asked him not to use any bleach. My husband passed gas and I smelled it and complained. He asked what was happening. He said that he used to be able to pass gas whenever he wanted to and I never smelled it. I told him that it was a side effect of one of the chemotherapy drugs, Cytoxan. Your sense of smell becomes keener. I told him that he wouldn't be able to put one over this nose again or at least until chemotherapy is through.

While I was on chemotherapy, I restricted myself from going any place where there was a large crowd. I did not go to church, since the flu season had peaked and I had no way of knowing what smell at church might start my upchucking. Instead, each Sunday morning I watched the televised service of a local Methodist church. It meant a lot to me at that time. My husband attended church as usual each Sunday.

When Monday morning came, I literally had to drag myself out of bed to go to work. Each day before I went to work I gave myself a subcutaneous injection of Neupogen and Procrit to keep my white blood cell count elevated and to increase the production of new red blood cells. My oncologist was keeping my white cell count increased up to 48,000 because of my profession. I work with biologically hazardous material. I wore a mask and protective gloves while examining all tissue specimens as usual. I wanted to be assured that I did not contract any infectious disease while my immune system was suppressed. Employees in the laboratory were told that if they had a cold, that they should wear a mask if they had reason to come to my office and speak with me about a technical problem. The co-workers and the employees of the facility were very protective of my health during this time.

I had been in the office only for two hours, when I received a phone call from a lady who was perturbed about the cause of her father's death. She requested an autopsy at the hospital where her father had been a patient, but the hospital would not perform one. She stated that her father had been dismissed from the hospital after being treated for pneumonia and that he had a history of chronic obstructive pulmonary disease, emphysema. He was transferred to hospice care after his hospitalization. He had been there less than six hours and was suddenly readmitted to the hospital and died. She begged me to do the autopsy. I told her that I really didn't feel much like it, because I had just started on chemotherapy last Friday for treatment of my breast cancer. I told also her that the procedure would be expensive. She said that she would pay. My staff did not want me to do the autopsy, but there was such a sense of urgency in this lady's voice, that I couldn't deny her and I reluctantly agreed to due the postmortem. She came to my office within thirty minutes after our phone conversation and paid both the hospital and professional fees. I performed the postmortem examination and was moderately fatigued at the completion of the examination. The autopsy was interesting in that the cause of the patient's death was a high-grade lung cancer that had not been diagnosed prior to his death.

Wednesday morning came. I ate breakfast and took my Glutamine, which was a supplement to prevent neuropathy (nerve damage) to my fingers and toes, which might be a toxic effect of the chemotherapy. It was a white tasteless powder, which I mixed with water and took in the morning and at night. It was only available at one pharmacy in the city.

When I arrived at work I was noticeably dragging. All of a sudden my co-workers were making me vanilla yogurt milk shakes. I had not weighed myself, but I guess I had scared everyone because within less than one week I had lost fifteen pounds. I guess that I had been vomiting more than I was eating. There was a possibility that I would need to have coverage. Another pathology group in the city was called. We met to discuss the type of coverage that I would need and they agreed to provide the coverage.

I increased my caloric intake substantially. Since I had been physically fit with a regular exercise program and maintained less than 5% body fat, it didn't take much to see why there was a dramatic loss in my weight. I increased my food consumption by increasing starch, protein and fat. I was now eating approximately 36 bagels a week. I added fried foods into my diet. I fried chicken wings and potatoes. I ate ten pounds of potatoes a week. I baked banana bread and cakes. One sheet cake was consumed every three days in my house and since my husband didn't care much about cake guess who was eating the majority of the cake.

My husband made me delicious fried mackerel and egg sandwiches on toasted bagels. I took two each day to work for lunch. I drank lots of Kool-Aid. Previously my preferred beverage was Coca Cola, but Coca Cola now had the taste of motor oil to me.

I was doing much better. I was able to determine that I could keep my food down if I vomited prior to eating. The food would then stay down and I would not be nauseous. I gained my weight back. My goal was to be at least seven pounds above my usual weight before my second round of chemotherapy.

My Hair! My Hair!

My hair had grown about an inch since my first treatment so I made a appointment with my stylist. He was as surprised as I was, that it had grown.

The next day I went to the oncology clinic for a check-up. They had received the results of my blood work and wanted to give me more Procrit in order to prepare for the next round of chemotherapy. They also gave me a brochure from The Wig Lady, a stylist who just opened up a shop for chemotherapy patients. I examined the brochure. The nurse and the receptionist had already picked out the ideal wig for me. They said this one looks just like your hair. I agreed with them, it did look just like my hair. I took the brochure with me and decided that I would call her for an appointment next week. I called her and left a voicemail message with my home phone number. Later that evening, she called. My husband was listening to our conversation even though he was acting like he was not. I made an appointment for Monday morning before work. On Sunday, I felt fine, so I decided to go to church. When I came back home I noticed a change in the texture of my hair. I didn't think much more about it though.

On Monday morning, when I awoke with my hair felt hard, dry and was matted in a clump. I looked in the mirror and saw that my hair in some areas was separated from my scalp. I got out my shears and started cutting the matted hair. I decided to where a hot rose pink African turban on my head, to hide the condition of my hair.

My husband and I prayed each day before work. This morning I felt as though he was making the prayer unusually long to interfere with the timing of my appointment.. When I left to get into my car, I told him that he had no right to make me late for my appointment and I further explained that I knew that he knew that I an appointment with The Wig Lady. He said that he was praying that I didn't lose my hair. I told him that I had already lost my hair and to look in the bathroom trash because a lot of it was there. I cried and left angrily.

I arrived at the Wig Lady's late but she did spend time with me. I was her first client. She told me that she decided to open the shop because she had a friend who was having chemotherapy and had lost her hair. They had gone to several shops looking for wigs and found that there was no privacy. They also went to the places where nonprofit organizations donated free wigs. The wigs were out in the open and no one fitted the patients. The quality of the wigs was also not good.

While I was in her shop I tried on several designer wigs with different styles, short bobs, straight bobs, curly bobs, and long and straight styles. I showed her a recent photograph of myself and pointed out the wig in the brochure that the nurse and receptionist of the oncology clinic had picked. She said, "It looks just like your hair!" We tried on a wig of that style. I ordered the wig and she said that it would be delivered to her shop in two days, Wednesday.

When I arrived at my office, everyone commented on the hot pink turban that adorned my head. I told the laboratory supervisor and the histology technicians that my hair would be totally gone by the end of the day. Five minutes later my office telephone rang. It was my husband. He apologized. He said he didn't know and that he had been praying that I would not lose my hair. I told him that I wished that I was not losing my hair also, but that this was the reality of chemotherapy. It kills all cells, good and bad. He asked me if I got my wig. I told him that I had ordered it and that I would have it on Wednesday.

When I arrived home later that evening, I took off my turban and began cutting the rest of my matted hair. I was now bald. I had not noticed that I also lost the few eyelashes and eyebrows that I had. My family members have scant eyebrows and eyelashes anyway.

I took off my suit and put on something more comfortable clothes to prepare dinner. My husband saw my bald head for the first time. He said, "You know what? You have a perfect bald head with no knobs, bumps or wrinkles?" He then rubbed my head for good luck. He said, "I'll call you my Gori Mapa." I asked him what did that mean and he told me, "Baldy, in Yoruba!"

Wednesday afternoon, the wig that I had ordered arrived. I went to the Wig Lady's shop to be fitted. It was a perfect color match with my natural hair. She trimmed the locks and cut the bangs to my desired length. I got a stand for the wig and also tried on some other styles that she had in the shop. I left the shop feeling good about the investment. There will never be another bad hair day for me.

I arrived home before my husband. I prepared the dinner, set the table and then looked at my new hair. My husband arrived. There were no pressing events during the evening. It took my husband two hours before he realized that I had a wig on. He said, "It really does look so much like your hair. I completely forgot that you had no hair. It doesn't really look like a wig."

Round Two

Friday came and I was ready for my next round of chemotherapy. When I arrived at the clinic, Dr. EE asked me how I was doing. He took my vital signs and performed a quick physical examination. He asked me if I had any problems. I told him that I had lost fifteen pounds and had everyone scared in the laboratory. I told him about how much I had to increase my caloric intake to weigh in seven pounds overweight. Dr EE told me that my laboratory work was acceptable and that I was ready for the next round of this fight.

I went to the infusion room where other patients were gathered.

My full entourage did not accompany me this time. I was no longer a rookie, but now a veteran. I made it through the first three weeks. I reclined in my chair and put up my feet. The nurse began the infusion. I greeted the other veterans in the room. I asked for the usual physician office magazines, Better Homes and Gardens, Times and Cosmo and was set for the next three and one half hours.

When the infusion was over, I put on my coat. It had started snowing. The white powder covered the parking lot. I walked slowly across the parking lot to the double glass doors of the hospital. The long corridors were darkened. I made my way to my office in the laboratory. I opened the door, entered my office and sat in my office chair.

It was 6:30 PM when I called my husband to pick me up. Within twenty minutes he arrived at my office. We walked to his white ML SUV. I climbed in on the passenger side and buckled up. I was hardly in the SUV two minutes when I had the pangs of nausea attack me. I told my husband to stop the vehicle immediately. I scampered out and vomited. He asked, "What's wrong?" I told him that it was the smell of the SUV. He said, "What do you mean the smell?" As I had mentioned before, one of the side effects of Cytoxan is that your sense of smell is extremely keen. I told him that it was the smell of the ceiling of the SUV. He told me that it was no different than my SUV and that I had driven it all week. I told him, "No! The vehicle is different." He said, "What do you want me to do? Do you want me to sell the SUV?" I told him, "No. You can't do that. It's a collector's item and the first ML to roll off the Mercedes assembly line in Alabama."

My husband had discovered one evening before he got in his ML to go home that there was a neon Mercedes emblem covering the entire hood of the SUV and that it was only visible under the parking lot lights at night. He had brought it home for me to see. He discovered from the dealership that the emblem was not visible during the day only at night and that it was put on the first two MLs that rolled off the assembly line in Alabama.

That weekend my husband cleaned the SUV and put Armor All on all the surfaces. He also put an air freshener in it. He asked me to sit in the SUV. I sat in the ML and told him that I could still smell the smell. He asked what I was smelling. I said the interior plastic. I told him to sit in my ML for fifteen minutes, smell it and relax. He stayed in my ML for fifteen minutes. When he stepped out, I told him to sit in his ML. He did as I requested and afterwards came out he said, "You are right. They do smell different." He asked again, "What do you want me to do?"I said, "Nothing. I just will not ride in your SUV until the chemotherapy is over."

Luckily, I had a three-day weekend. I had coverage for the pathology department for Monday so that I could recuperate and go to work on Tuesday when I was sure I wouldn't be dragging. I tried to drink a Coca-Cola. I still was no longer able to drink it. It still tasted like motor oil. Kool-Aid was now my drink of choice instead. I looked at my hands and noticed that there were brown-black streaks on my fingernails. I looked at my feet and my toenails showed similar changes. I looked at my tongue in the mirror, it also had black streaks on the right side and in the middle. My stomach began to feel hot and acidic. I then I vomited and was in no discomfort.

When I went to work my colleagues also noticed my nails and that they were discolored and darkened. One physician and colleague during a meeting kept staring at my nails. He later asked, "Are you going Gothic on us?" I told him that it was a side effect of the chemotherapy and that my toenails are also affected. I showed him my tongue. I told him that they will get a lot darker with each round of chemotherapy and so will my skin tone before it is over.

Round Three

I arrived at the clinic. Dr. EE. performed his usual examination. He noticed that my nails were black brown, a lot darker since Monday. I told him, "Just wait until you see my tongue." When he saw it, he said, "I usually see patients with some darkening of the nails, but not to this extent and your tongue and its black streaks... It looks like you are going to show more toxicities." My laboratory work was fine and blood pressure normal. I weighed in now ten pounds over my ideal weight. Maybe I've been eating too well. I told Dr. EE that the Glutamine was not working and that I had noticed a slight numbness of my fingertips and toes and that I had doubled the amount of Glutamine that I was taking, but it was just not working.

I went into the infusion room, where the other veterans were sitting. I reclined the chair. The nurse started the infusion. I would be there another three and one half hours. After the nurse started the infusion she left and went to use the telephone. The nurse called the pharmacy, the sole provider for Glutamine in the area. She asked the main pharmacist what type of Glutamine he had, the name of the manufacturer, the container size and amount. She then called the manufacturer and spoke with a representative and told her that a physician patient stated that the Glutamine was not working, despite the fact that she had been taking twice the recommended dosage. The representative asked whether or not I was taking the Glutamine with oxidizers. The nurse said that the type of Glutamine stocked by the pharmacy did not mention oxidizers. The pharmacist had told the nurse that this was the same Glutamine that they had stocked for the last three years. The representative asked her to tell them the name of the pharmacy and its location. She said that the pharmacy did not order the Glutamine with oxidizers. She said that she would notify the pharmacist and rush Glutamine with oxidizers to the pharmacy.

The nurse came back and reported to me what had transpired and said that I should be able to get the Glutamine with oxidizers on Monday. This means that none of the patients who received the Glutamine for the last three years complained. They had accepted the neuropathy or didn't understand their signs and symptoms as what was supposed to be an expected toxicity. If a doctor states that this drug is preventative for the neuropathy or nerve damage that may develop from the chemotherapy and the drug doesn't work, the doctor should be told that it is not working.

I thanked the nurse for the phone calls she made. I was thankful that I would be able to get the correct Glutamine. It would not be fun having numb fingers and toes and not knowing where my feet are when I'm walking. Numbness is definitely not a good thing.

When the infusion was over, I went to my office to close up. My husband picked me up. I told him about the great discovery of the day. I was glad I had another three-day weekend, even though I would be recuperating. Five more rounds to go and only one more round of nausea left.

I picked up the Glutamine with oxidizers. It consisted of a white powder with brown and red powdered flecks. When the powder was mixed with warm water it turned red and looked and tasted much like tomato soup. This was far more palatable than the tasteless white powder.

The creases in the skin of the palms of my hands and the soles of my feet were very dark. The rest of my skin tone was very dark brown, almost black. My husband had been complaining that he could smell the chemotherapy drugs when I sweated and urinated. I did not doubt that he could because I could smell them and I had an exceptional good sense of smell at this time because of the Cytoxan.

I met one of the patients on whom I had recently made a diagnosis of breast cancer. She came to ask me what the next step was. I referred her to Dr. EE's office. She became a patient of his partner. She began chemotherapy shortly after me. She was only able to complete the third round because her physician feared than if she continued, she would have more nerve damage because of a previous existing condition. Many times patients are not able to complete the full course of treatment. I guess I should consider myself blessed.

Soon it would be Thanksgiving Day. Some of my out of town relatives, in-laws, wanted to come for the holiday, but I was in no mood for company. My husband stalled them off. They were not aware of the fact that I was sick. The workweek was short because of the Holiday and I thanked God.

When Thanksgiving Day arrived I was determined to cook a full Thanksgiving Dinner for two. When I awoke that morning at 5:30 AM. I prepared and seasoned the fourteen-pound turkey and set the oven for 325 degrees. I opened the dry yeast packets and added the warm water, salt, oil, and sugar to a large bowl. I later added flour to the mixture and stirred. I covered it with a saran wrap and waited for the dough to rise. I later started slicing and dicing the vegetables for my rice dressing.

For the first time I found that my legs were weak and tired. I never had to sit down while preparing the Thanksgiving dinner in my entire life. I can only imagine that this is may have been the type of tiredness that my Mother may have felt her entire life. She had been crippled with rheumatoid arthritis when I was two years old and never verbally complained about the disease. I only heard an occasional sigh. Her weakness and tiredness showed however in her eyes. Now I was the one who was working slowly and my legs were very weak.

I turned on the water and scrubbed the outer surface of the sweet potatoes, and put them in a large waterless cookware pot to let them cook so that I could peel and slice them later to prepare the candied yams. I sauteed the vegetables for the rice dressing and put rice in the rice cooker. I washed and peeled apples for the apple pie and arrived at a point where I could sit down to complete the rest of my peeling, slicing and dicing.

Normally, when I prepared Thanksgiving Dinner I would start at 5:30 AM and have the dinner with baked rolls, rice dressing, roasted turkey, vegetables, cranberry sauce, apple and sweet potato pies and carrot cake completed by 1:00 PM. This time Thanksgiving dinner was served at 8:00 PM. We gave God the praise and thanks!

Round Four

The nails of my toes and the skin of the soles of my feet were thickened. Reddened and painful spots began to appear on my toes and on my soles. I showed Dr. EE, who examined the soles of my feet prior to the administration of the last round of Cytoxan and Adriamycin. This was a side effect of the chemotherapy. There was no increased numbness of my fingers and toes. The Glutamine with oxidizers seemed to be working.

My vital signs were taken and I was escorted to the infusion room. A patient came in to be seen. Dr. EE and the nurse saw her, then they sent her to me. The nurse said, "This patient came in to show us her fingernails. We told her that they usually do not get very dark. She asked us what was the darkest they can get, so we thought we would introduce her to you." I recognized the name of the patient. I had diagnosed her breast cancer less than two months ago. I showed her my fingernails, and my toenails and my tongue. I told her that this wasn't usual and that most patients do not develop pigmentation to this extent.

The patient smiled and told me thanks and then left the clinic. The nurse then cleaned my port and accessed it to begin the infusion. The sticks to access the port were still painful each time. I guess that I'll never get used to that. I reclined my chair and decided to sleep today since I was the only patient present and being infused. Four hours later the infusion was complete. I walked across the parking lot with my sore feet. I got into my car and went home for the weekend. Only four more round to go.

Over the course of the next two weeks my feet began to feel like I was walking on sand paper. The red splotches were very painful. The palms of my hands looked like they were rough and looked dirty since they were dark brown with patches of thickening or hyperkeratosis. The one flat wart that I had on the back of my right hand began to enlarge and I began to have began to have multiple warts on the backs of both hands. The largest and unsightly ones, I chemically treated.

Christmas was coming soon. I at least needed to go out and get something for my husband despite my weakness. Maybe, I'll get out this weekend.

Round Five

I have made it through the first four rounds of chemotherapy. Glory be to God who has seen me through thus far! It was only through Him that my health was brought to my attention. My husband one day during morning prayer in August prior to the biopsy of the mass under my arm had asked God, "Why there? Why under her arm?" The immediate response that he heard was, "It was only place that I could safely put it to bring it to her attention!" My husband didn't understand, but I fully knew what was meant by it. The chances of breast cancer having contralateral axillary metastases (or spread of the tumor to lymph nodes under the opposite arm) are less than 1%. How it occurs without evidence of spread of the cancer to some other site in the body is a bone fide miracle.

Dr. EE examined me again. Although I still felt like I was walking on sandpaper, the purple lesions on my feet were not as painful as they had been during the previous two weeks. The laboratory work was satisfactory.

We discussed the next four rounds of chemotherapy. I would be given one drug, Taxol. I was told that the drug was suspended in castor oil. Knowing my clinical history of being allergic to soybean oil, several other allergens and clinical hypersentivity vasculitis, Dr. EE was not going to take any chances with me. He certainly did not want me to have an anaphylactic, allergic reaction in which my blood pressure bottomed out and I stopped breathing. He decided to administer intravenous Prednisone first and then start the infusion of Taxol. My blood pressure would be monitored every five minutes for the first fifteen minutes, then every fifteen minutes for the next hour and then every half hour. I went to the infusion room and reclined in the chair. The nurse said that this infusion would not be as long. That's good. I can get home early, I thought. The nurse accessed the port and started the infusion of the Prednisone. She then prepared the Taxol, which was pink liquid suspended in oil. She put a blood pressure cuff on my left leg above the knee and obtained my blood pressure. After the infusion of the Prednisone was complete she started the infusion of the Taxol. During the first fifteen minutes of the infusion she kept close watch of me asking if I was doing okay. I replied that I was fine. She later took my blood pressure every fifteen minutes for the first hour and later every half hour.

I had no complications during the infusion, but after the infusion I could smell the Taxol in my sinuses. It had the very distinct medicinal smell of castor oil. I can still remember the taste and smell of castor oil when I was an adolescent. I was given white powdered cascara in orange juice for bowel prep. It has tasted so bitter that after that experience, I did not drink orange juice for the next twenty years.

I felt somewhat waterlogged, whether or not it was from the knowledge that I would be retaining water from the Prednisone administered to me or if it was a fact, I could not say. When the infusion was complete, I went back to the hospital and closed my office for the night. My husband picked me up this time because we didn't know how I would be feeling after this infusion. He asked me how I was and I answered, "Just fine. I have this funny smell in my sinuses though." He asked if I felt nauseous. I replied, "Surprisingly no!"

The weekend came and I had no nausea. I went to Sunday morning services. I saw a fellow breast cancer survivor. I had not seen her in six months. She updated me with her projects on nutrition at the university. Her mother had recently died and there had been some problems with the settlement of her estate. She said that you never really know your siblings until the death of a parent. It was nice seeing her again. I went directly to the grocery store after our conversation. It felt good to go to the store again and not to not feel nauseous while shopping. It was an unseasonably warm day in January and the birds were out singing and giving thanks to God. I am just as thankful for the beautiful day as I am for being alive. I later drove around enjoying the sights for a half hour after leaving the grocery store. I was getting hungry and headed for home.

At 3:00 PM, exactly 48 hours after completion of my infusion of Taxol, I began to feel spontaneous sporadic shooting pains in different areas of my extremities. An hour later, I had pain all over my entire body. It was constant and unrelenting. My husband asked me what was wrong and I told him that I was in extreme pain. I hadn't experienced anything like this before and he knew that I could usually suppress pain on my own. He asked where I was hurting and I told him that I was hurting all over my entire body, every muscle, every nerve. He reached out and touched me and I said, "Don't touch me!"

I went to the bathroom medicine cabinet and found a few pain tablets of Tylenol with codeine, Tylenol #3. I took one tablet, swallowed it, drank a glass of water and went to bed. I awoke later in the evening and got something to eat afterwards, I took another tablet and went back to bed. I awoke in time for the 10 o'clock news and the weekly sports review on television. I later went back to bed again. I sighed, "God, if I am not going to make it through, take me now!"

My husband decided to declare it a night. He went upstairs. I was glad, because any movement of the bed or my body just exasperated the pain. He had been sleeping upstairs mostly and I downstairs because, he could not stand the smell of the chemotherapy on my body.

Luckily, I still was taking Monday off after my treatments. When Tuesday came, I was still in pain. It was like my nerve endings were on fire. I was unable to predict when a shooting pain would go down my extremities. It was intermittent and unrelenting. It even hurt to comb my hair.

Tuesday afternoon I decided to get a slightly stronger medication. I definitely did not want to ask for one, but I felt that I had to so that I could function during the rest of the week. I went to the clinic and was given some sample medications, enough to get through the rest of my treatments. The medication worked fine. I took only half the recommended amount, because I didn't like the side effects of pain medications. Unfortunately, I experienced the major side effect constipation.

By Thursday I was definitely plugged up. I had not had a bowel movement in three days. I had been given a stool softener, Ducolax and had been taking it daily. I went to the clinic on Friday, still no relief. My abdomen was slightly distended and I was extremely uncomfortable. I went to the clinic again. The nurse said, "Still no relief?" I said, "None yet!" She said, "Well drink plenty of water. You should have a bowel movement pretty soon."

Now I know how the elderly feel when they come to the doctor with a chief complaint of no bowel movement. That seems to be one of the most important complaints in that age group and now I have the same complaint. I left the clinic and returned to the hospital to close my office for the day. I went to the grocery store to pick up a few things for dinner.

While I was standing in the long check-out line, I suddenly felt the urge. I kept waiting in line, checked out and felt that I could make it home. My husband opened the door. When I arrived I didn't speak a word of greeting I just rushed to the bathroom to relieve myself. What a welcomed explosion!

Round Six

Friday has come, five treatments down and only three more to go. I completed my work in surgical pathology and left to go for my treatment. The walk across the parking lot was somewhat refreshing. It was beginning to snow. When the automatic doors opened, a cold blustering wind chilled me to the bone. I neglected to take my scarf with me and I kept thinking, "God, please don't let my wig blow off." The wind was so forceful that when I began to run it lifted my feet off the ground. I became airborne and bumped into a pole.

I made it across the parking lot and opened the clinic door. I stamped the snow off my shoes. I had to be extremely careful not to slip in the doorway. As I entered the office, the receptionist said, "I guess I don't need to ask if it's cold, snowy and the wind is blowing!" I nodded in assent. I went into the exam room where the nurse was waiting. She took my vital signs and then Dr. EE entered the room. The nurse told him that after today's treatment that I will only have two treatments left. He said jokingly, "I looked over the charts yesterday and I know that she has at least five more treatments left!" I told him, "No, the nurse is right. After this treatment, I have only two more left, thank God. It looks like I am going to get through this.

Dr. EE examined me and looked over the laboratory work that had been just faxed. Everything was in order so I went to the infusion room for the sixth infusion and my second round of Taxol.

Mr. M, a 35 year old patient who had a high-grade lymphoma, tumor of the lymphatic system, was being infused. I have seen his weight decrease over that last two months. He has had a second relapse. At least my tumor seemed to be responding to the treatment appropriately. The nurse brought me the newest issues of Better Homes and Garden and Cosmo. I thanked her.

Dr. JP walked into the clinic to ask me a question about another patient's results. I told him what he needed to know. He had a new surgical female resident accompanying him. He asked how I was doing and I told him that I was doing fine. I reclined in the chair and got ready for my infusion. I knew what to expect now with this medication and I knew what I had to do to cope with the side effects. No complications were noted during the infusion. After the infusion was completed, I scampered across the parking lot. It was still snowing. The wind had died down in the past few hours though. I returned to my office, called my husband and told him that I was on my way home and closed shop for the weekend.

Round Seven

My husband told me that we were going to have company this weekend, my brother-in-law, James. My husband did not tell any of his family members anything about my physical condition. My husband wanted to keep it a secret. It was also the week of my birthday. Luckily, I get along well with my brother-in-law. He is not much of a bother. I cook the food and he eats it and gets more food for himself whenever he wants. He even knows where the snacks are kept. My husband had brought a new car home, a Mercedes SLK. He told me to pick up his brother from the airport and to later tell him what I thought of the vehicle.

I went to the airport to pick up James. The little black sports car performed right on the mark. It was exhilarating. James was standing right at the front door of the airport so I didn't have to bother about finding a place to park or get out of the car into the cold and then pay unwelcomed parking fees. I honked at him and he saw me. I popped open the trunk and he put his briefcase in it. I asked him how he was doing, he said that he was fine and so was the wife and kids. He asked about the vehicle. I told him that his brother had brought it home and asked me to see what I thought about it.

I told him that this was the first time that I had ever driven it and that I definitely liked it and that I didn't want to give it up. When we arrived home my husband met us at the gate. I scurried inside, hung up my coat and went to the kitchen to prepare dinner. While I was working my husband and his brother went upstairs and conversed until I called them to dinner. I could tell by James's eyes that my husband had told him about my condition. I showed him my nail changes and my tongue and told him that I had no hair and that I was now my husband's Little Gori Mapa. He laughed when I told him. I told him that I was okay and that I was making it through my last rounds of chemotherapy now.

My husband said the dinner prayer. We were definitely glad to see James again. After dinner I retired early, to get ready for the long day. I would have another round of chemotherapy tomorrow afternoon. I said my goodnight.

Friday afternoon again and round seven was uneventful. I parked the car in front of the clinic since it was becoming dark earlier. After the infusion I got into my vehicle and went home. When I arrived, I found to my delight that my husband had already prepared dinner. I ate and help with the dishes. I conversed with my brother-in-law for about and hour and then retired early. TGIF and the weekend!

When Sunday morning came my brother-in-law and I went to church together. My husband went to an earlier mass. I had prepared most of Sunday's dinner on Saturday evening, so that Sunday would definitely be a day of rest. When we arrived home, we called James' s wife and children; I told them that we would probably see them soon.

I prepared the table for dinner. During dinner, my husband and

James reflected on things that happened during their childhood. My husband as a teen used to try to get out of the house without his little brother James tagging along. He would constantly look over his shoulder to see if he was being followed and at every step there was a little shadow scurrying behind a tree or an opened a door each time he would look back. After several blocks he would call him and they would walk side by side. I can remember similar times with my siblings.

I prepared the dessert. I had just finished scooping up the ice cream when I began to feel shooting pains down my leg. I told my husband and his brother that I was going to bed. It was exactly 48 hrs from the last Taxol infusion. I took my pain medication and retired for the evening.

Round Eight

I am so thankful that I have made it to this last round and it is not a bit too soon. Unfortunately, it had been more difficult for me to remain a compliant patient. The daily Procrit and Neupogen injections for twelve days after receipt of the chemotherapy had become seven to ten days of injections, simply because I had convinced myself that I didn't need that many injections. I did not like the taste in my mouth, nor the medicinal smells after I gave myself an injection. Whether it was a true smell or only psychological, it didn't seem to matter to me. I was just tired of being a good patient. I was tired of being stuck each week for lab work. My skilled laboratory staff had done a great work by being able to get blood from a turnip. They managed to find the only accessible vein that I had and to access it for blood. The vein on right thumb held up well, being stuck twice a week and and was still accessible after seven rounds of chemotherapy. I thank God for this. It for me was much better than having the Port accessed for the laboratory tests. Accessing the port to me was psychologically more traumatic.

I arrived at the clinic for my last round of chemotherapy, weighing in at 155 pounds. This is the most that I had ever weighed in my entire life thanks to the Prednisone. My laboratory tests results were acceptable. I told the nurse about my non-compliance as a patient and that I was elated that this was the last round. She was also happy for me. She said she was glad that I came to the clinic and followed through with the treatment plan, because she now knew that I was going to make it now. I told her that I knew that she knew and that I had seen what she had seen also, just by looking at photographs that had been taken of me in the recent past.

Dr. EE was seeing another patient and her husband about a recent pathology test. It was not good news. When the patient went to the infusion room for another round of chemotherapy, Dr. EE introduced her to me. He told her that I was going to receive my last round of chemotherapy for breast cancer and that I was the pathologist at the hospital. I spoke with her for a while. I told her that the treatment is one step and a time and one day and a time and that I was pulling for her and that I would pray for her. She smiled and said, "Thank you. I'll pray for you too!"

I reclined my chair for what I knew would be the last infusion and decided to sleep for the next three hours. God has been good to me and He is not through with me yet, no not yet.

Lessons To Be Learned
1) Know the physicians who will be treating you.
2) Know what your treatment plan is.
3) Know the stage of you disease.
4) Know your pathology diagnosis and obtain a copy of the pathology report and go over it with your physician.
5) If chemotherapy is part of your treatment plan know the drugs that will be administered , why they are given and the side effects of each drug.
6) If you are nauseated, ask for medication to treat the nausea.
7) You do not have to be in pain during your treatment, if you need medication, ask for it.
8) Know who the contact person is while you are undergoing treatment, so that you can ask questions and get help when you need it.

RADIATION

It was a cold winter day with blustery winds and an overcast sky. I chose to receive my radiation treatment in the suburbs. The medical center was approximately a thirty-minute commute by interstate from my office. Dr. GW, the radiation oncologist who belongs to the same group as Dr. EE, was my treating physician. I knew and trusted the members of this group. The scheduling for my radiation treatment would be a little more flexible for me, given the time constraints of my occupation. Getting out to see the terrain would also be beneficial and a form of relaxation for me.

When I arrived, the receptionist greeted me. I didn't have to fill out mounds of paper because my records were automatically transferred to the clinic. The nursing assistant showed me the locker room. I disrobed from the waist up and put on a gown. I was escorted to one of the examining rooms where a nurse took a limited history, my vital signs and weighed me in. I was told that Dr. GW would be in shortly.

I was glad to see Dr. GW. He is a prince of a man, sensitive and caring. I am grateful that he referred me to a female radiologist for my additional diagnostic studies last September. Dr. GW conducted a thorough examination. He told me that he intended to treat the following areas: left breast surgery site, complete right breast, right axilla, and both supraclavicular areas (above the collar bone near the neck). An additional radiation boost would be given to the right back and scapular area)right upper back). The treatment was a little more extensive than usual, but one has to consider what is known. The tumor presented as metastases or spread of tumor underneath the right arm. Biopsies of the right breast however, showed no evidence of tumor. Usually a malignancy of the right breast metastasizes to the right axilla lymph nodes (under arm lymph nodes). What we know about my case is that we have a documented tumor in the left breast, which is 8 mm and had been surgically removed and no tumor in the right breast that can be documented. Spread of a tumor from the left breast to the right axilla is something that occurs in less than 1% of breast malignancies. It is highly possible that there may be an occult tumor in the right breast that is not visible by mammography. This is why the both breasts were going to be treated even though the tumor in the left breast and the right axilla were similar in appearance when examined under the microscope.

I was sent to radiology for a chest x-ray and a CT scan of the chest. This study together with other views taken by the radiation therapy department would be used to determine where the exact coordinates where the radiation treatment would be directed and to make sure that heart, and most of the lung tissue are shielded from the radiation. Radiation treatment was slightly more extensive in my case. Only one breast and/or axilla usually receives treatment in most cases. My case is a little more challenging for the radiologic technicians in determining the ports under Dr. GW's guidance. Computer technology has changed treatment plans dramatically since I first entered medical school.

After the CT was completed a few additional shots were taken in the department, I was told to come back tthe next day and be ready for a more extensive process setting up the coordinates and to be prepared to be tattooed.

I drove back to the office to complete my work and later drove home. I told my husband and my sister Cynthia what had transpired. She said that she would like to go with me sometime. I told her that she could come on Thursday or Friday since tomorrow would take two to three hours. She said okay.

I went to work the next morning and told my co-workers of my experience. I also told them that I thought this process would be a piece of cake compared to what I had previously been through. The only thing that I might have to worry about is whether or not my skin integrity could hold up and whether or not my wig falls off during the procedure. I also told them that I had to leave earlier today since the process would be a little more extensive, setting up the coordinates for the radiation. I told them that I would be back in three hours.

I drove to the center and was greeted by Glenda, the receptionist as I entered. I looked at the films with the technicians. The first thing they said to me was, "Didn't you tell us you were allergic to some types of metal?" I told them, "Yes?" They showed me my right axillary films with an abundance of metal clips. I said, "That's just great I hope it doesn't cause any problems. My body might decide to expel each one out on its own. I have enough skin problems and I hope this doesn't become a source for more.

I then went into the treatment room. I was introduced to two radiologic technicians whom I would see daily. One technician was familiar face to me because he also worked at the medical center where a worked.

A partial body cast was made for my upper torso with my arms resting above my head. The material used was very cool. The cast later hardened into a perfect mold of my upper torso. It was to be used each day so that my body would be in the same position during treatment. The technicians started setting the coordinates. The process was tedious. One technician marked my skin with a marker. He told me not to wash off the marks that night, because I would be tattooed the next day.

When I arrived the next day, I expressed my concerns because I didn't want a permanently tattooed torso. I asked how big this tattoo is going to be. The technician told me that the actual marks were minute black-blue pinpoint marks that would hardly be noticeable. He was right. They were hardly noticeable and each pin prick tattoo mark made did not hurt as much as I had thought that it might. But I knew that I will not be receiving any other tattoos just for the fun of it. The complete process took about an hour. The technician made certain that each coordinate matched up with the coordinates that had been determined the prior day.

When the process was complete, I drove back to my office. I talked to my histotechnician and told her what had transpired and revealed one of the small tattoo marks. I later completed my work and drove home. When I arrived my husband was very much interested in seeing my tattoo. I showed it to him. He was as surprised as I was, because it was much smaller than he had expected. I told him the first treatment would be tomorrow and that Cynthia had requested to come along to find out what it was like.

The next day, I left the hospital 45 minutes earlier so that I could pick up my sister and then head toward the center. My sister was as talkative as usual. The 30-minute trip seemed a lot shorter with her aboard. When we arrived at the clinic, I introduced her to Dr. GW. I told him that she wanted to see what they do as far as cancer treatment. Dr. GW took her to different areas of the facility, so that she could see what radiation treatments were all about. I went in for my first treatment, which should only last ten to fifteen minutes.

I disrobed and went to the radiation treatment room. The

technician immediately placed my form on the table. I placed my body in the form. The technician aligned and centered my tattoo marks with appropriate coordinates and began the treatment. The treatment was given to the left lumpectomy site, the right breast and the right axilla and the supraclavicular areas (areas on each side of the neck above the collar bone). When the treatment was complete, I was in no discomfort. It was quick and I was ready to go. When my sister arrived, she explained to me everything that Dr. GW had shown her. She quite was enthusiastic and I was glad that I approved of her going along for the trip. We thanked everyone and told them to have a good weekend.

When we got to the car, I asked my sister whether or not she wanted to go to the shopping center on the way home. She consented and we shopped for three hours. We tried on clothes and shoes and looked at the sales on costume jewelry. She bought a skirt and a couple of sweaters. I bought a couple of sweaters also. I usually buy suits, but not this time. I have enough suits in my already packed closet, which needs to be cleaned out.I need to assess what I haven't worn in the past year. After shopping I took my sister home. I thanked her for going with me. It was good for the both of us.

Every Monday through Friday I drove to the radiation center for treatments. I saw the changes in the seasons. When I first started my trips the grassland was brown. Sporadically the roads became sprinkled with snow and I would have to wonder whether or not black ice was forming over the bridges. The ride for the most part had been peaceful. I watched as buds began to appear on the trees and as the grasslands and the barren fields began to sprout green. One day when I arrived at the center, Glenda, the receptionist asked me to come back outside. She said that she wanted to show me something. She took me to one of the topiaries near the front door next to the circle drive-thru and pulled back the tree limbs exposing a nest containing four featherless baby wrens. She said that this was the second year that the mother had chose to put her nest there. I looked at the babies, new life on this earth, while me and others like me are fighting to stay alive on this earth. It is well and life springs anew each and every day. Take the time to notice and see the wonders of each and every day. See God makes all things new! The promise of new life!

My treatments were going well. I managed to keep my skin

integrity and made sure that I applied lotion to my chest every morning and every night. The technicians and Dr. GW felt that I would probably be able to complete my treatment without a complication. I had only three more treatments to go when I developed a dime size superficial erosion of the skin of my right breast. I told the nurse and Dr. GW examined the erosion. He said, "We have to stop the treatments for a week." I told him, "Okay, no problem." I applied creams to my chest very liberally at night during the entire treatment as I had been told. During the next week, all of the skin on my chest behaved like sunburn and began to weep and become scaly and peel. This continued to the end of the week. When the next Monday came I called Dr. GW and told him that I felt I needed another week to heal. He said no problem and that he would see me in a week. The next week when I arrived at the center, Dr. GW examined me. He said, "Well, it looks like we can proceed with the last three days of the treatment." I was glad. The last three treatments went without any complications. The entire radiation treatment went better for me than the chemotherapy. I did not experience any tiredness, I had no anemia. My only complication was the skin erosion and sun burn scaling rash. There was a slight increased firmness of both breasts. They were similar firmness to my thighs. My radiation treatment was finally over. I was given a graduation certificate of completion of my treatment plan. Thanks be to God I made it through!

Lessons To Be Learned
1) Discuss your treatment plan with your radiation oncologist.
2) Be sure to ask questions.
3) Know your contact person if you should experience an complications.
4) Know what the adverse effects of treatment may be.
5) Learn how to care for your skin during treatment.

ANTI-ESTROGEN THERAPY

I made an appointment to see Dr. EE who prescribed Tamoxifen (a selective estrogen modulator which blocks the estrogen receptors) for anti-estrogen therapy. I thought that the cessation of Premarin was tough, but once I started taking Tamoxifen, I soon found out that I was mistaken. The hot flashes were now more frequent and more prolonged. I had a fan in my office and one in the gross examination room and also one in the post mortem examination room, the morgue. The temperature in the morgue is usually maintained at 60 degrees Fahrenheit, but I still needed the fan.

At home I had a small fan in the kitchen, one by my chair in the living room, one by my bathroom vanity and one on my nightstand. My nightgown was soaked by mid-morning. I ate ice chips for relief. My husband told me that he could tell when I was flashing while I was sleeping, because my covers would fly off and then later when he looked my covers would be back on, while I was still asleep. I don't think he realized however, how many times I got up in the middle of the night to get ice and water, nor was he aware that I would awake at 3:30 AM and not be able to go back to sleep, because of the hot flashes. I contacted Dr. GW who gave me samples of Effexor to treat the hot flashes. It worked extremely well. After 48 hours I gave him a call because I all of a sudden felt like there was a metal plate in my head separating my right brain from my left. I felt like one side of my brain could not communicate with the other. Dr. GW told me to get off the Effexor. I discontinued it.

When my husband wanted to have sex, I soon found out that I had extreme vaginal tightness and dryness. The next day I was prescribed an estrogen vaginal cream for use as needed. My husband also began complaining that my body and urine had a funny smell because of the Tamoxifen. He also discontinued the Tamoxifen. He prescribed Arimidex. I found it to be less harsh than the Tamoxifen, but much more expensive. Less than 2 months later, my husband complained of the smell of the Arimidex also. I consulted the Dr. EE, the oncologist again and this time he prescribed Femara. I was also prescribed Raloxifene to prevent osteoporosis (bone loss from the lack of estrogen). I was able to take these drugs without any complaints from my husband. I continued these expensive drugs for the next five years. I restarted my exercise regimen and lost the weight I gained during chemotherapy. I have been disease free and have had no disease recurrence.

Lessons To Be Learned

1) If your tumor is estrogen receptor positive be sure to ask your physician about anti-estrogen therapies.
2) If you experience side effects, notify your physician who may suggest alternative drug or therapy.
3) Do not be afraid to discuss with your physician things that effect your quality of life or life as you knew it before treatment. Your physician may be able to help you.

BREAST HEALTH PRIMER

BREAST ANATOMY

The breast or mammary gland is situated between the superficial and deep fat of the skin. The function of the mammary gland or breast is for lactation or the production of milk. The breast goes through many changes in its development. At birth some infants have a slight increase of breast tissue due to the mother's hormones. The breasts of some infants may secrete a milky substance. These changes may only last from three to four weeks. At childhood there may be some branching of the ducts or gland units.

Figure 12.1.

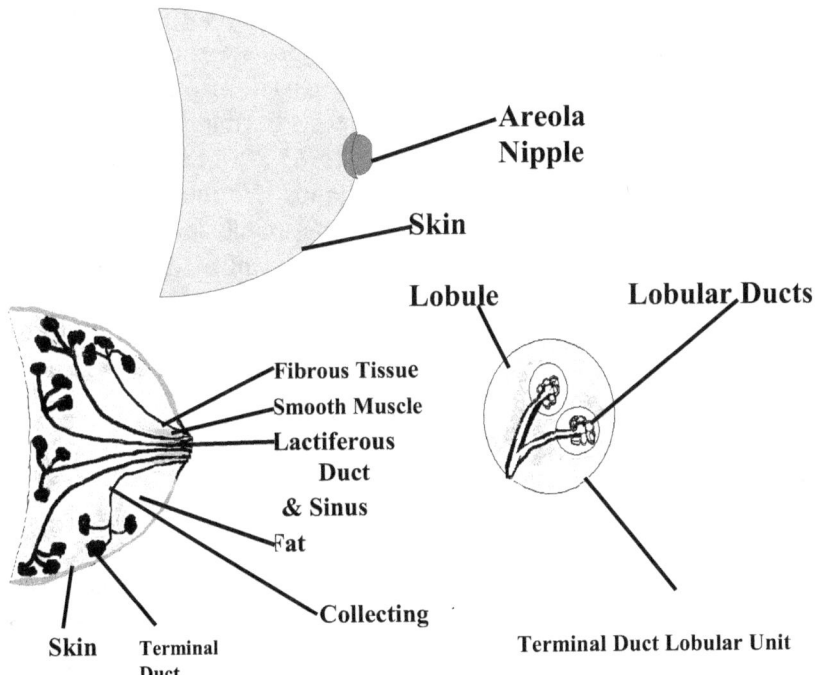

There are no significant changes of the breast during childhood. The skin of the nipple and the skin surrounding the nipple, the areola is pigmented. This pigmentation increases during puberty and adolescence when breast growth is stimulated by estrogen. During puberty and adolescence the greatest changes that take place in the female breast due to the hormonal changes. The pituitary gland secretes Follicle Stimulating Hormone (FSH) which stimulates the ovary follicles or eggs to produce the hormone estrogen. Prior to ovulation the estrogen hormone levels exceed progesterone hormone levels, but after ovulation progesterone hormone levels exceed estrogen hormone levels. Estrogen and progesterone stimulate the growth of the breast tissue. The breast bud or primitive duct or gland begins to bud and branch to form a unit or duct system. The breast or mammary gland duct system consists of ducts (tubules or glands), fibrous connective (supporting) tissue and adipose tissue (fat). The breast undergoes cyclic changes during each menstrual cycle. These changes occur both in the breast ducts and the supporting stroma of the breast. Some secretory activity or secretions are seen in the breast ducts, but these changes are mild. The supporting tissue may have some edema or may be seen as slight swelling of the breasts during the cycle.

The mammary gland is divided into 15 to 20 lobules or units. Each lobule (unit) consists of smaller ducts (glands or tubules) called lobular ducts, which produce secretions or fluid. The lobular ducts are connected to larger collecting ducts and the lactiferous (milk) ducts and sinuses (dilated sacs), which have openings extending into nipple. The nipple is located in the center of the duct complex. The nipple area has abundant sensory nerve endings. The nipple is elevated above the level of and surrounded by the areola (the pigmented area of the skin surrounding the nipple). The nipple has ducts, nerves and smooth muscle fibers, which contract to compress the ducts, and make the nipple erect.

During pregnancy estrogen levels are high and significant changes in the breast occur. The breast cells increase in number. There is a overgrowth of the glands which exhibit marked secretory activity and have distended lumens or openings. The glands begin to produce milk. During menopause the breast atrophies or involutes, losing glands and increasing in fat. The supporting tissue of the breast becomes more fibrous. Involution is a process which happens over time and during that time changes in the consistency and firmness of the breast can be noted.

The breast has a lymphatic drainage or vessels, which play a role in how malignant breast cancer spreads. The breast gland has central, lateral and medial networks of lymphatic vessels or channels, which drain into the lymph nodes in the axilla or underarm area (75% to 98% of the channels) or to the internal mammary lymph nodes in the chest (5% to 25% channels). The lymphatic channels drain into the lymph nodes. The breast also has a venous drainage to groups of veins under the arm and in the chest which contribute to breast cancers' ability to spread to the lung, liver, bone and brain.

Lessons To Be Learned

1) The breast or mammary gland develops under the stimulation of hormones, estrogen and progesterone. These hormones are essential in the development of the ducts system or gland unit.
2) The breast undergoes cyclic changes with each menstrual period.
3) The breast undergoes functional changes to produce milk.
4) The breast at menopause begins to atrophy or diminishes in size and gland prominence.

BREAST SELF EXAMINATION

Know your breasts! The American Cancer Society no longer recommends that women should perform a Breast Self Examination (BSE) when a patient reaches 20 years of age. BSE is considered optional by the American Cancer Society. More recent scientific literature has questioned the value of the examination and it has now become acceptable for women to choose for themselves how often they will perform BSE or whether or not they will perform BSE at all. [1, 2] There are studies that suggest that BSE is a benefit at all ages, but other studies suggest that BSE alone does not reduce the mortality or deaths from breast cancer and that it may cause harm by unnecessary biopsies. [3]

Intensive instruction on BSE does not reduce the mortality or numbers of those dying from breast cancer.[4] As a physician and breast cancer survivor, I encourage you to be as healthy as you can be and be aware of your own body especially your breasts. Breast cancer is the second leading cause of death of women in the United States and there is still a role for breast self-examination. Mammography does not pick up every breast cancer and up to 43% of breast cancers are detected by a palpable mass on examination of the breasts and are more likely palpable in women who do not undergo yearly mammography screening.[5] If you choose to perform BSE, that is your choice to do so. Know your body! Breast cancers may be detected when they are smaller and at an earlier stage among women who practice BSE.

You should acquaint yourself with the normal anatomy of your breasts and if there are any changes in their appearance or a mass or lump is felt, schedule an appointment with your health care professional or physician. If you are a mother or an older sister who routinely performs monthly breast self- examinations you should teach your daughter or your sister the technique of BSE before adolescence, so that they can know what is normal.

If you choose to perform the Breast Self Examination (BSE) it should be performed about one week after the start of your period or after the normal monthly swelling of your breasts resides. BSE can be performed at regular or irregular intervals. The purpose periodic breast self exams is to promote breast awareness. The examination is performed in front of the mirror disrobing from the waste up. Look at your breasts with your hands raised over your head. Observe the appearance of your breasts in the mirror. Are your breasts the same size and shape? Are there any skin changes (i.e. redness, rashes, weeping, difference skin texture, firmness or hardness)?

Look at your nipples. Are the nipples normally everted (stuck out) or inverted (stuck in)? Most nipples are everted. Inverted nipples occur in less than 10% of females. A normal everted nipple that becomes inverted is not normal. Notice whether your nipples are symmetrical (the same) or if there is a pull, dimpling or folding of the skin or area of retraction of the skin. Look at the breasts with your hands raised over your head. Repeat the same examination with your hands on your hips and then with the palm of your hands pressed together.

Examine your breasts in the shower and later while lying down with you arm behind your head and placed on a pillow. Examine each breast with the free hand either **in an up and down, wedge or circular pattern**, until the entire breast has been examined, using your three middle fingers, flatly pressing the breast and feeling for lumps or nodules. After one breast has been examined, place the opposite arm behind your head and examine the other breast. It does not matter whether you use the up and down, circular or wedge pattern to examine your breasts. Either technique is fine as long as you work from the outer aspects of your breasts to the nipple area. If you notice a nipple discharge or fluid while examining one part of the breast be sure to notice what part of the breast you were examining while this occurred. Pinch the nipples and look for any discharge or material that can be expressed from them.

Figure 13.1

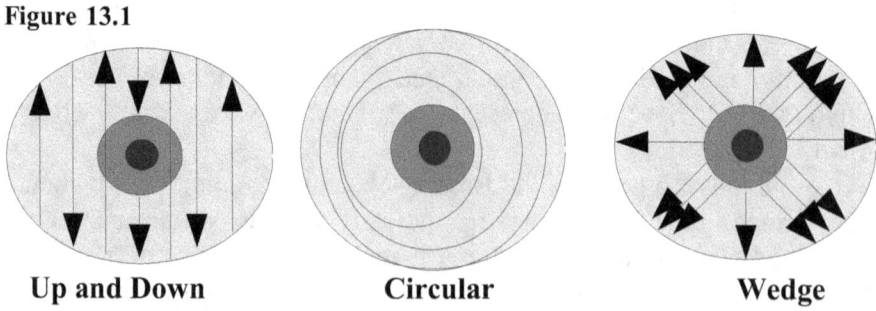

Up and Down   **Circular**   **Wedge**

Check both underarms for nodules, masses or enlarged lymph nodes.

If you have any questions on what you are feeling or how a normal breast should feel, contact your physician, a local health care facility or the American Cancer Society. They may have examination models and or recorded CDs or tapes for you to use or offer education classes about breast self-examination. If when performing your breast self examination any part is abnormal, or if you find a lump, nipple discharge or skin changes, promptly schedule an appointment with your physician. If you find anything at all you should not procrastinate. Do not think that what you find will necessarily go away. Make an appointment with your physician. An examination by your physician is imperative as well as a diagnostic mammography examination or and other tests if so ordered by your physician.

How-be-it rare, juvenile breast cancers may occur and can be discovered by breast self-examination. The youngest case of breast cancer I have seen was in a six year-old boy. When his family physician asked his parents how long the tumor or mass had been there, they said one month. The boy shook his head and replied a year. The family physician was more inclined to believe the boy because of the size of the tumor and believed that the parents had ignored the tumor and procrastinated getting their child the medical care that he needed.

Know your breasts! Know what is normal, so that if you discover a subtle change or area of concern in your breasts you can schedule an appointment with your healthcare professional as soon as possible. If you are younger than 40 years of age your physician or other health care professional should perform a breast examination at least every three years and recommend mammography based on your risk. If you are a woman who is at high risk for breast cancer, then your provider may recommend screening mammography earlier, age twenty-five or thirty depending on the risk. Your physician may decide to schedule examinations and mammograms more frequently depending on your clinical risks and family history.

The US Preventative Services Task Force (USPSTF) revised its recommendations for breast cancer screening in 2009. The USPSTF did not recommend routine mammography screening for the 40 to 49 age groups based on the lower cost effectiveness screening in this age group. for regular mammography screening. Many experts and groups have wondered whether or not this was a cost cutting or health care rationing issue by the government especially since the National Cancer Institute published a monogram showing the benefits of breast cancer screening mammogaphy in women age 40 to 49 years or age. The National Institutes of Health (NIH) also has advocated more research to explore the areas where there is considerable health disparities (differences between breast cancer rates, risks and survival in Blacks, Whites, Native Americans, Asians and Hispanics and the barriers that exist to screening mammography, delays to diagnosis and treatment). The USPSTF 2009 recommendations are as follows:

- Regular mammography every 2 years from 50 to 74 years of age
- Routine mammography screening from age 40 to 49 not recommended and should be based on individual risk
- There is insufficient evidence to suggest that screening mammography should be extended beyond 75 years of age
- There is insufficient evidence to recommend clinical breast examination (CBE) in women forty years and older
- Evidence does not support teaching women breast self examination (BSE) as a screening tool

The American Cancer Society (ACS), the American College of Radiology and the American College of Obstetricians and Gynecologists are recommending that physicians and patients continue to follow the ACS guidelines below:

- Annual mammograms starting at age 40 years and continuing as long as a woman is in good health

For individuals of normal risk the current recommendations are at age 40 years a clinical examination should be performed by your healthcare professional every year. The current recommendations are that mammography should begin at age 40 and be performed every year. Screening mammography is the best test a women can have to prevent or reduce her risk from dying from breast cancer. Screening mammography can be started earlier than age 40 years and should also be based on the woman's risk for breast cancer. There is no such thing as being too old for regular mammography. Regular screening mammography in women over 80 years of age has shown to improve 5-year survival rates.[6] Keep track of your health insurance policy benefits. Your insurance should cover cost of mammography. If you are uninsured, help is available. Contact your local American Cancer Society or Susan G. Komen Foundation or the Y-Me National Breast Cancer Organization, and other charitable local agencies. They should be able to direct you to clinics and services that are funded or they may have access to funds to provide screening mammography at little or no cost to you.

References:

1. The American Cancer Society (ACS) annual guidelines for the early detection of cancer.January/February issue of CA Cancer Journal Clinic.
2. Barclay, Laurie and Nghiem, Hien T., American Cancer Society Annual Guidelines for Early Cancer Detection, CA Cancer Journal Clinic Jan/Feb 2006
3. Kosters JP, Gotzschke P "Regular self-examination or clinical examination for early detection of breast cancer (Review)" *Cochrane Database Syst Rev* 2008; 3:DOI: 10.1002/14651858.CD003373.
4. Thomas DB; Gao DL ; Ray RM ; Wang WW ; Allison CJ et al. "Randomized Trial of breast self examination in Shanghai: Final Results., J National Cancer Inst. 2002; 94(19):1445-57.
5. Degnim AC. Palpable breast cancers are more common in women not undergoing annual mammography. Journal of the Am College of Surgeons, March 2010.
6. Badgwell B, et al. Mammography before diagnosis among women age 80 years and older with breast cancer. J Clin Oncol 2008; DOI 10.1200/JCO.2007.12.8058

Lessons To Be Learned

1) Breast self examination (BSE) has not been proven to be effective.
2) Whether you decide to perform BSE is considered optional, but you should familiarize yourself with what the normal breast feels like.
3) If you want to learn BSE contact your physician or your local American Cancer Society.
4) Regular screening mammography should begin at age 40 years or earlier based upon the woman's breast cancer risk.

KNOWING YOUR BREAST CANCER RISKS

Be in the know! The risk factors for developing breast cancer in a person's lifetime or at a young age include factors of the family history and genetic factors. High risk genes account for less than 5% of the breast cancer diagnoses. Approximately 60% of breast cancers occur in the absence of any known risk factors and for most women lifestyle factors like childbearing, the use of hormone replacement therapy, obesity and alcohol consumption are the greatest risks. Do you have factors that put you at an increased for breast cancer? The following list is a summary of known risk factors.

BREAST CANCER RISK FACTORS
- Family history of breast cancer in all first degree maternal and fraternal relatives (i.e. mother, sisters or daughters, father, brothers or sons)
- Family history of high risk genes or cancer syndromes:
    - Hereditary Breast Ovarian Cancer Syndrome BRCA1/BRCA2
    - CHEK2 gene - 1100delC cancer gene
    - Li Fraumeni Syndrome, p53 gene
    - Cowden's Disease, Hereditary PTEN Syndrome
    - Peutz Jegher's STK11 gene (Intestinal Polyposis)
    - Hereditary Diffuse Gastric Cancer, CDH1 gene
- History of Ovarian cancer, fallopian tube cancer or cancer of the abdominal cavity
- Late childbearing age
- Early puberty and menarche (menses)
- Long-term use of hormone replacement therapy
- Oral contraceptives (birth control pills)
- Childbearing in late age or lack of childbearing
- Moderate to high alcohol consumption
- Ionizing radiation of the thorax or chest (as in Hodgkin's lymphoma)
- Obesity and sedentary lifestyle
- Late menopause
- Postmenopausal hormonal replacement therapy
- Early onset breast cancer

- Multifocal or bilateral breast disease in yourself or a family member
- Relatives with male breast cancer
- Family history of non-breast malignancies, (i.e. ovary, prostate, cervix and non-melanoma skin cancer)
- History of benign breast disease
- History of atypical hyperplasia/LCIS/DCIS and situ carcinoma [1]
- Prior history of breast cancer
- High breast density

Benign (non-cancerous) breast disease has an associated breast cancer relative risk of 1.6. For women 50 years of age and older there is a slightly increased relative risk of 1.95. For families with no history of breast cancer the risk ratio is 1.32. Patients with a weak family history have a risk ratio of 2.12 and those with a strong family history 2.19. **Only 5 to 10% of all breast cancers are due to inherited mutated genes and high risk genes are detected in less than 5% of newly diagnosed cancers.** Up to 60% of breast cancers occur without any known risk factors.

It is known that patients with relatives who have had breast cancer have an increased risk for the disease. The risk increases with increasing numbers of affected relatives and the decreasing age of the family members affected. Women with only one first degree relative diagnosed with breast cancer before age fifty are not at increased risk for developing breast cancer in early life.

INCREASED RISK FOR DEVELOPING BREAST CANCER YOUNGER <30 YRS	
	Hazard Ratio
Two cases of female breast cancer in first-degree relatives	3.09
Two cases of female breast cancer in first or second-degree relatives < 50 yrs	3.36
One case of female breast cancer < 40 yrs in a first- or second-degree relative	2.06
Any case of bilateral breast cancer	3.47

The **risk for being diagnosed with breast cancer at 30 years of age or less** is increased in the following incidences:
- At least two first degree relatives with breast cancer
- At least two cases of first or second degree relatives under age fifty with breast cancer
- At least one case of female breast cancer under age forty in a first or second degree relative
- Any case of bilateral breast cancer.[2,3]

Families with a history of the **Breast Cancer Antigen, (BRCA1 and BRCA2)** gene mutations have a predicted risk. These gene mutations are most common in women of Ashkenazi Jewish descent. For a patient with the BRCA1 gene mutation located on chromosome 17, the risk for developing breast cancer by age 70 is 45-87% and the risk for developing ovarian cancer is 16-63%. BRCA1 breast cancers are usually of worse prognosis. They are high grade cancers. 90% are Estrogen receptor (ER) negative and HER2 receptor negative. These tumors usually spread hematogenously (through blood vessels) instead of lymphatic channels and vessels thus making them more aggressive. The BRCA1 gene is also associated with an increased risk of cancers from colon, pancreas, stomach, and fallopian tube. BRCA1 tumors are more aggressive that BCRA2 tumors.

The BRCA2 gene mutation is located on chromosome 13. It is associated with an increased risk of cancer of the breast, ovary, colon, esophagus, pancreas, stomach, hematopoetic (blood cells), prostate and malignant melanoma (cancer of the pigment cells of the skin). The risk of developing breast cancer by age 70 is 26- 84% and the risk of developing ovarian cancer by age 70 years is from 10-27%. BCRA2 breast cancers are usually of moderate grade, ER positive and Her2 negative. [4]

It is important that you know that the risks for breast cancer are increased for women with early onset breast cancer regardless of the status of the BRCA gene in the family. In women with a history of breast cancer who have prophylactic mastectomies (removal of the breast to prevent cancer), some 11.1% of the mastectomy specimens (breasts removed) may have occult (hidden) malignancies or cancers. Approximately 57% of these malignancies have been invasive cancers (tumors spreading outside that are not confined to the breast ducts or have spread outside the breast ducts) when compared with similar specimens from BCRA positive patients. [5] For women who had been previously diagnosed with cancer and elected to have a prophylactic contralateral mastectomy (removal of the other breast to prevent cancer) in a study at the University of Texas MD Anderson Cancer Center an occult malignancy or hidden cancer was found in the contralateral or opposite breast in 5 to 15% of patients. The tumors in the contralateral breasts had moderate to high risk histopathology changes (disease changes) in the breast tissue when examined under the microscope.[6]

There are other gene mutations that are associated with an increase risk of breast cancer. CHEK2 is an 110delC germ line gene mutation and is associated with a two-fold risk increase in the development of breast cancer over the general population. The mutation of the p53 gene on chromosome 13 is known as Li-Fraumeni syndrome. It is associated with an increased risk of premenopausal breast cancers, childhood sarcomas, brain tumors, leukemias, lymphomas(tumors of the lymphatic system) and adrenal gland cancers. Crowden's syndrome is a mutation on the PTEN gene, chromosome 10q23. The risk of breast cancer is 25 to 50%. [7]

It is important to be aware that there are hereditary risks of breast cancer and to be informed. The presence of early onset disease in a family member may denote hereditary cancer. Multifocal (multiple breast cancers) and/or bilateral disease(disease in both breasts) may be indicative of a genetic risk. The fraternal (father) history of the family is just as important and the maternal (mother) history since there is a fraternal risk of transmission. Male breast cancers although uncommon do occur and may indicate disease which is inherited. The association of other malignancies, namely prostate, cervix and melanoma skin cancers is a definite hereditary risk factor for breast cancer.

Genetic counseling is strongly suggested for hereditary breast cancer. Issues such as privacy rights and quality of life should be discussed to help allay anxiety and help you make informed decisions. A genetic counselor can also guide you in the decision making process as to whether or not expensive genetic testing in needed. If you happen to have one of the cancer genes (BRCA1/BRCA2, CHEK2 or others), unaffected family members should be tested so that health care options can be discussed with family members that may have the gene.

Modifying the Risks

Women who have the BRCA1/2 breast cancer genes have a four fold increased risk for breast cancer occurring in the contralateral or opposite breast compared to women who are not carriers of the mutant gene.[8] Women who develop breast cancer before age 55 have a 20% probability of developing cancer in the contralateral breast, while women who do not carry the BRCA1/2 gene have a 3% risk. Women carrying the BRCA1/2 gene have a lifetime breast cancer risk of 36% to 84%. Prevention strategies in high risk women can aid in preventing up to 1500 cases of breast cancer per 100,000 and prevention strategies for low risk women can prevent up to 25 cases of breast cancer per 100,000.

Affected family members and carriers of the BRCA1/2 gene mutation because of breast cancer risk may elect to have bilateral mastectomies. This can reduce the risk of breast cancer by 90% or more. However, risk reducing mastectomy in BRCA1/2 mutations carriers with a history of cancer in one breast does not necessarily result in improved survival.[9] The overall survival for mastectomy and non-mastectomy groups is about the same. Breast conserving therapy with or without radiation therapy can be an effective short term option.[10] Chemotherapy ovarian oblation to eliminate the ovaries ability to make estrogen and progesterone or the surgical removal of the ovaries are also options as a prevention strategies to reduce breast cancer recurrence.

Chemoprevention, the administration of selective estrogen receptor (ER) modulator drugs, like **Tamoxifen** may be a good choice for some patients and used to prevent breast cancer. **Tamoxifen** has been found to offer anj overall 50% reduction of breast cancer risk. **Aromatase inhibitors (AIs)** inhibit the enzyme aromatase which is needed for the body to make estrogen and have a similar affect as Tamoxifen in reducing breast cancer risk. The **AIs** also have been shown to be less toxic in postmenopausal females. The common drug **Aspirin** has been found to significantly reduce the risk of in situ estrogen receptor positive breast cancer but not overall risk of invasive cancers.[8] Other factors which may help to modify your breast cancer risk include maintaining a normal weight, having a early first pregnancy, breast feeding and the delay of the onset of early menses.

Family members with the BCRA1/2 genes may elect to have removal of both ovaries and fallopian tubes to prevent ovarian carcinoma. This procedure reduces the risk of ovarian cancer by 95%. However, similar tumors develop in the abdominal cavity in 4.3% of patients who have had both ovaries and fallopian tubes removed some 20 years after the procedure. The surgical procedure, however, is favored, since the ovarian cancers that usually develop are high-grade tumors and aggressive. There are no good screening tests for ovarian carcinoma, although the blood test CA-125 has been used as a screening tool as well as transvaginal ultrasound imaging. The results of studies using oral contraceptives to prevent ovarian carcinoma have been inconsistent.

Eight out of nine women who develop breast cancer do not have an affected first degree relative. Most women who develop breast cancer develop it after age fifty. The lifetime incidence of breast cancer is 5.5% for women with one affected first degree relative and 13.3% for women with two affected first-degree relatives. [11,12] Your knowledge of your family history is extremely important. It is imperative that you know your family history and your genetic predisposition for the disease. You should not assume that the cancers that may occur in your family are just sporadic.

Knowing your risks and your family history will help your doctor determine how often you will be examined and the frequency of mammographic examinations and other tests that your physician may order. It will determine whether gene cancer tests or the breast cancer antigen tests, BRCA1 and BRCA2 and CHEK2 should be ordered and whether a genetic consultation requested is requested by your provider. Discuss your concerns about genetic testing with your physician. Please note that some who are at increase risk for breast cancer never develop breast cancer. At present we do not know who will not develop the disease, but in the future we may be able to determine this.

References:

1.Wickerham, D.L. Paik, S. et al, Journal Natl Cancer Institute 2004, April; 96(8)pp.616-20

2. deBock, GH, Jacobi, et al; A Family History of Breast Cancer Will Not Predict Female Early Onset Breast Cancer in a Population-based setting. BMC Cancer 2008:, 8:203.

3. Czyzewski, Andrew, Family History Poorly Predicts early Breast Cancer, BMC Cancer 2008:203.

4. Bernan, DB et al (1996). A common mutation in BCRA2 that predisposes to a variety of cancers is found in both Jewish Ashkenazi and Non-Jewish individuals. Cancer Res 56:3409-3414.

5. Feldman E, et al The incidence of occult malignancy and atypical histopathology in prophylactic mastectomy specimens after uninformative BRCA testing ASBS Meeting 2008.

6. Lehman CD, Gatsonis C, Kuhl CK, et al. MRI evaluation of the contralateral breast in women with recently diagnosed breast cancer. *N Engl J Med*. 2007;356(13):1295-1303.

7. Auger, Danielle, The Genetic Link to Breast Cancer, Advance News Magazine for Administrators of the Laboratory, Oct 23, 2006. p 1-9.

8. Gierach GL, et al Nonsteroidal anti-inflammatory drugs and breast cancer risk in the National Institutes of Health-AARP Diet and Health Study Breast Cancer Res 2008.

9. Heemskerk-Gerritsen BAM, et al. "Is risk-reducing mastectomy in BRCA1/2 mutation carriers with a history of unilateral breast cancer beneficial with respect to distant disease free survival and overall survival?" EBCC 2010; Abstract 500.

10. Pierce, l etal. "Local therapy options in BRCA1/2 carriers with operable breast cancer: the importance of adjuvant chemotherapy: EBCC 2010; Abstract 7N.

11. Wang Jiping J., Constantino, J. et al., J Natl Cancer Inst 2004 Apr; 96(8)616-208 PG, 2004.

12. Biostatistical Center, National Surgical Breast and Bowel Project of Department of Biostatistics, Graduate School of Public Health, University of Pittsburgh, Pittsburgh, PA 15213, USA.

Lessons To Be Learned

1) Assess your breast cancer risks by knowing your family history for breast cancer, breast cancer genes and for non-breast cancers (ovary, prostate, cervix and non-melanoma skin cancers).
2) Assess your lifestyle risks for breast cancer (birth control pills, hormone replacement therapy, obesity, alcohol use, sedentary lifestyle, previous chest radiation, history of breast disease, early menses, late first pregnancy and late menopause).
3) Discuss your risks for breast cancer with your physician.
4) The risks for breast cancer are increased for women with early onset breast cancer regardless of the status of the BRCA gene in the family.
5) The maternal and fraternal family history of breast cancer are equally important in determining the risk for breast cancer.

THE MAMMOGRAM

Mammography is a low dose x-ray imaging used for examination of the breasts. It is a screening test for the early detection of breast cancer and currently one of the most effective ways to detect breast cancer. It is the suitable screening tests for most women who are not high risk for breast cancer. About 20% of women are at high risk for the disease and other additional tests like ultrasound and MRI (magnetic resonance imaging) may be needed to detect breast cancer.

When breast cancer is detected early, it is most curable and can be treated by simple lumpectomy (excision or surgical removal of the lump) or breast conserving surgery (BCS). **Early detection is the most important key to survival**.

Racial disparities in breast cancer survival rates still exist in the United States. The 5 year survival rate for breast cancer for White patients compared to Black patients is 14% higher and it is also higher than in Hispanics. [1] Other disparities that exist are that Black women may have to wait twice as long as White women to be given a definitive diagnosis of breast cancer, may also wait twice as long to begin treatment after the diagnosis[2] and may be offered a mastectomy instead of breast conserving surgery (BCS). The availability of mammography and education for all ethnic groups are key in eliminating some of the disparities in treatment and in early detection. More is being done to address these and other disparities in treatment and health care access.

Mammography use of women in their 40s has stagnated somewhat and women without insurance are more likely to not undergo mammography screening.[3] Mammography is the most important test that a woman can undergo to reduce the chance of dying from breast cancer. It is highly recommended that women who are 40 years of age or older begin mammography screening as recommended by your physician based on your risk assessment for the early detection of breast cancer.[4] The individual assessment is based upon family history, genetic risk and the presence of the BRCA1/2 gene or other mutant genes, and other risks. Women ages 50 to 74 years should have mammography performed at least every two years. .

Two-thirds of women do not follow the recommended screening guidelines. Lack of insurance should not be an excuse for not getting a mammogram. Organizations like the American Cancer Society, your local Medical Society, the Susan G. Komen Foundation, the Y-Me National Breast Cancer Organization or other local charitable organizations can either provide assistance or recommend resources for you so that you can get the study done for free or at minimal cost.

The mammogram can show changes in the breast up to two years before a tumor is clinically apparent. The mammogram cannot detect all breast cancers and positive changes (changes suspicious for cancer). Not all changes suspicious for cancer on a mammogram are cancer. Slightly less than one-fourth of such lesions detected by mammography are cancer.

Before having a mammogram, you should discuss with your physician any signs, or symptoms or problems that you may be having with your breasts. The best time to schedule your examination is the week after your period. Make sure that the place where you will have your mammogram is certified by the American College of Radiology (ACR).

On the day that the examination is scheduled do not wear deodorant, talcum powder or lotion, which may appear, as calcium spots on the x-ray. Completely fill out the clinical history sheet and discuss any problems with the technician. If you have a suspicion that you are pregnant, tell the technician. If you have breasts implants be sure that facility you use has experience working with patients with implants. If you have had any prior mammograms at a different facility, be sure to make arrangements for the prior films to be sent to the radiologist at the facility where you are getting your mammogram so that he or she can compare the previous films with the present.

Be sure to ask when your results will be available and call your physician for the results. You do not want to be the patient with an abnormal mammogram and nobody called you back or looked at your results to see if you needed additional studies. Keep track of your results.

Mammograms can miss up to 15% of cancers in breasts that are highly dense and lesions that may be too small to be detected. It is possible to have a tumor that cannot be visualized by conventional mammography.[4] If you have abnormal symptoms that persist after a normal mammogram, it is up to you to bring the issue up to your physician and ask if any other tests that can helpful. Additional tests like ultrasound or MRI may be required in up to 15% of mammograms.

The mammography unit is a machine with a platform on which the breast is placed. During the mammography the technician assists you in positioning the breast in the unit. There is a cone like device or paddle made out of Plexiglas above the platform. It compresses and spreads the breast tissue. It also holds it in place while top to bottom and oblique views are taken.

Conventional film or screening mammography is ordered in women with no signs or symptoms of breast abnormalities, and usually only the top to bottom and oblique views are taken to detect abnormalities. Diagnostic mammography is used to investigate a patient with clinical abnormalities or suspicious areas of the breasts and/or skin, pain or changes in the nipple, breast discharge or a breast mass. The radiologist may order additional views during the procedure.

You may feel pressure during the procedure. The sensitivity of each individual to the procedure is different. Aspirin, Ibuprofen or Tylenol can be taken an hour before the procedure to ease the discomfort of the

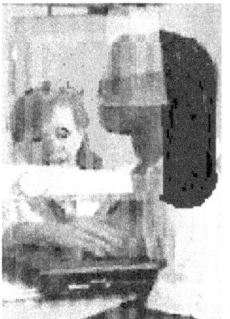

Figure 15.1

examination. Lidocaine gel may also be used during the study to ease discomfort. If the compression is very uncomfortable, alert the technician.

Full-field digital mammography is a method, which rapidly replacing x-ray film. Solid-state detectors convert x-rays into electric signals similar to the technology in digital cameras. These images can be seen on a computer screen, printed and saved. The digital images can easily be retrieved to compare the images with previous examinations. Computer aided detection (CAD) uses a digitized image of a mammogram or digital mammogram to highlight images to alert the radiologist that further studies may be needed. The above methods are comparable to mammograms and have been found to be better in detecting breast cancer in premenopausal and perimenopausal women who have dense breasts.

The American Cancer Society recommends for women of average risk regular yearly mammography after age 40 and a clinical breast examination (CBE). Women who have a lifetime risk for breast cancer greater than 20% or a strong family history for breast or ovarian cancer or previous history of atypical hyperplasia, carcinoma in situ or extremely dense breasts should have screening at shorter intervals. Screening magnetic resonance imaging (MRI) is recommended in these individuals.[3]

The recommendations are early detection by yearly mammography and clinical breast examinations or other studies suggested by your physician. Do not procrastinate in having your examination. The proportion of women aged 40 years having both a mammogram and clinical breast examination is 51% for insured women, and for uninsured women is 28.2%. Women with inadequate insurance are at a higher risk of dying from breast cancer. African American women are at a 64% higher risk of dying from breast cancer than white Americans. As I stated before, lack of insurance should not be an excuse for not having a mammographic examination. There are charitable organizations that will pay for a mammogram or offer it at a reduced. Contact your physician or local Cancer Society, the Susan G. Komen foundation, or local Medical Society for names of organizations that can assist you. Routine clinical breast examinations and mammography are a matter of health and an important key to staying healthy, alive and well.

Lessons To Be Learned

1) Regular mammography exams as recommended by your physician based on your risk assessment from you family history, genetic risk, the presence of BRCA1/2 and/or other mutant genes, obesity and other lifestyle factors is necessary for early detection of breast cancer.

2) Mammography can reduce the chances of dying from breast cancer.

References:

1. Coleman MP, et al "Cancer survival in five continents: a worldwide population-based study (CONCORD)" *Lancet Oncol* 2008; DOI: 10.1016/ S1470-2045(08)70179-7.
2. MedlinePlus Health Information; "Black women wait longer for breast cancer diagnosis, treatment"; April 22, 2010.
http://www.nlm.nih.gov/medlineplus/news/fullstory_97930.html
3.Miller JW et al. "Mammography Use from 2000 to 2006: State-level trends with corresponding breast cancer incidence rates"; Am J Roentgenol. 2010; 192(2):352-60.
4. Lie, D.; Medscape Family Medicine. Cases in disparity" Breast Cancer screening: How to guide Black, White, and Asian patients. March 3, 2010.
5. MayoClinic.com, Tools for healthier lives. Mammography X-ray exam *to detect breast cancer. Oct 7, 2005.*
6. Saslow, D., Boetes, C. et al, Cancer J. Clin, 2007; 57(2)75-89. American Cancer Society guideline for breast screening as an adjunct to mammography.
7. Radiology Info, The mammogram, RSNA, September 26, 2005. p. 1-4.

UNDERSTANDING WHAT'S NEXT!

This year in the United States despite the fact that breast cancer incidence rates have recently declined by 8%, invasive breast cancer will still be diagnosed in slightly over 175,000 to 200,000 women. Approximately 12%, one of every eight, women will develop invasive breast cancer in her lifetime. Breast cancer is the second leading cause of death in women in the United States. Approximately 15% of the diagnosed total cases of breast cancer, 62,000 cases, will be non-invasive breast cancer (breast cancer confined to the breast ducts) or carcinoma in situ (CIS). The remaining breast cancers will be invasive cancers. Breast cancer can also occur in men and approximately 1,700 will be diagnosed this year. Male breast cancer represents approximately 1% of the cases that will be diagnosed. Approximately 40,000 deaths will occur this year from breast cancer.

Screening mammography is still recommended for breast cancer screening and is the most important test a woman can undergo to reduce her chances of dying. November 2009 the United States Preventive Services Task Force (USPSTF) issued guidelines recommending biennial screening mammography to start at age 50. This is in stark contrast to the recommendations of the American College of Radiology (ACR) and the Society of Breast Imaging (SBI) who recommend that women with an average risk of developing breast cancer start screening mammography at age 40.[1]

For high risk individuals a mammogram and annual MRI is recommended starting at age 30. High risk individuals are:

- ◆ Carriers of the BRCA1 or BRCA2, CHEK2, PTEN or p53 mutation genes
- ◆ Individuals who are untested and have a first degree relative with a BCRCA 1 or 2 , CHEK2, PTEN or p53 mutation genes
- ◆ Those with a high lifetime risk of greater than 20% for breast cancer i.e. history of previous thoracic or chest radiation, atypical duct hyperplasia (abnormal or pre-cancerous changes of the breast duct cells), a previous history of breast cancer and highly dense breasts.

Ultrasound and MRI are adjuncts or additional tests used for diagnosing breast cancer. Newer technologies for diagnosis and treatment have been developed in the last 25 years. Digital mammography was developed to increase the accuracy of mammographic screening, offering an improvement over film mammography by easier access to images, computer assisted diagnosis, improved image storage and retrieval and lower radiation dosage. It is especially useful in the examination of dense breasts in women 40 to 50 years of age. It has been found to be superior to conventional mammography, and is less expensive than MRI but not as good .[2] MRI has been found to be cost effective in women with BCRA1 between the ages of 35 to 54 years but is generally not cost effective for BRCA2 carriers.[3] MRI can more effectively rule out minute invasive cancers. It can be used to detect small proliferative changes (changes with an increase of breast ducts or glands) and in non-invasive cancer or ductal carcinoma in situ (DCIS), cancer that has not spread outside the ducts. Another investigational tool that may help distinguish between benign and malignant (cancerous and non-cancerous) breast lesions is that of optical tomography which measures the hemoglobin content of breast masses. When used with mammography and ultrasound this technique may give a more accurate preoperative diagnosis.[4]

Mammogram Report

The results of a mammogram report can either be normal or abnormal. If you receive a report that your mammogram is normal and your health care provider or physician has found no abnormalities on examination and you
haven't found anything abnormal on your breast self examinations, there is no reason to worry. Continue with your BSEs, clinical breast examinations by your provider and life as usual. Make sure that if you do find an abnormality before your next scheduled examination or mammogram, that you contact your physician for an appointment as soon as possible. Do not worry that your physician may dismiss your complaint and think that you are a hypochondriac. Don't cause yourself needless anxiety and don't procrastinate. Your health care provider knows that despite the fact that your examination may have been normal a few months ago, things can change. Any new breast complaint, a mass, a skin rash, a nipple discharge or anything suggestive of malignancy should

receive a thorough evaluation. [5]

If you find an abnormality by BSE, and the clinical breast exam by your physician and mammogram are normal, your health care provider will probably repeat the clinical breast examination, go over your clinical history and re-evaluate your risk factors. Depending on your risk factors your physician may suggest re-evaluation within 2 months since changes felt by BSE may be normal physiologic changes.

Physiologic changes can occasionally create suspicious densities on mammogram. I have personally seen a few cases where a suspicious densities by mammography were nonexistent on repeat exams and I have known several cases where patients had been scheduled for needle localization of their masses prior to surgery only to find that their masses had disappeared. This resulted in the cancellation of surgery.

Mammography fails to detect approximately 15% of palpable malignant or cancerous tumors, your doctor may decide to order a diagnostic mammography with magnification or additional study in the area or suspicion. An ultrasound can also helpful to further evaluate and localize the lesion, but this too has its shortcomings. An MRI may also be valuable in detecting a non-palpable lesion.

If you have a change by BSE and the mammogram shows a discrete mass. Your physician will probably refer you to a surgeon or radiologist who can obtain core needle biopsies (cylindrical tissue biopsies obtained with a needle) of the breast mass. The core needle biopsy is a minimally invasive procedure and the initial optimal choice for sampling radiologic (X-ray) image detected abnormalities of the breast. Since 75% of the abnormalities detected by mammography will be invariably benign or non-cancerous, skilled surgeons, radiologists and pathologists reached a consensus in 2005 that physicians should attempt to replace traditional invasive procedures with less invasive diagnostic methods, like needle biopsies of the breast and biopsy of the sentinel lymph node, the lymph node closest to the breast in the axilla or underarm area.[6] Since minimal invasive needle biopsy procedures are the optimal choice, open surgical biopsies are unnecessary in the initial evaluation. Suspicious areas of concern by mammography, i.e. calcifications or lumps can be localized and biopsied using a needle. The entire area of concern may be removed if needed using this procedure.

Fine needle aspiration (a sampling of the cellular material by drawing it into a needle attached to a syringe) can be done for confirmation of malignancy or cancer in larger masses or tumors. A radiologist, a surgeon or a pathologist may perform this procedure. Ultrasound may be used to localize and view the lesion if it is not readily palpable, then the needle is stuck into the lesion or mass. [7] The doctor will insert a needle into the mass and pull back on the syringe to aspirate or suck material into the hub of the needle on the syringe. If the mass is cystic the syringe may be filled with fluid which may be yellow and watery or brown yellow with some streaks of blood in it. If the mass is solid then no fluid will be noted. Slides are usually prepared using the material acquired. The slides and material are sent to the laboratory or prepared on site for examination by the pathologist. The pathologist may be asked to confirm that the material is acceptable, prior to your leaving the procedure room in case an additional aspiration is needed. A week or two after the aspiration your physician may ask you to make an appointment for a second visit to determine what additional procedures may be necessary or to see if the mass has resolved or completely disappeared.

If a non-discrete or irregular nodularity or thickening of the breast tissue is noted by clinical breast examination and a density or lesion or mass is present by mammography, an open surgical biopsy may be requested. Statistically, if a woman is premenopausal the result of such a biopsy is more likely to be a benign or non-cancerous or normal physiologic change. Cysts account for 25% of new breast lumps in premenopausal women and less than 1% of cystic lesions may have an underlying tumor. The risks of cancer in a new breast lump is 1 in 10 women. Cancer is of higher incidence in postmenopausal women but it can occur in premenopausal women as well. All breast complaints must be evaluated. If woman is postmenopausal there may be more concern for malignancy, since most cancers occur in postmenopausal women. In either case, you can be reassured and satisfied that your doctor or health care provider will thoroughly evaluate and address your symptoms so that the diagnosis is not missed and so that there is no delay in diagnosis.

If a definite mass is noted by the clinical breast examination and by mammography, it is imperative that the mass be evaluated by needle core biopsy or open biopsy. If you have a breast mass do not delay in obtaining a diagnosis. There should be no delay in obtaining the diagnosis of the breast mass. Make sure you that you are scheduled for a biopsy as soon as possible. Again biopsies can be easily obtained by inserting a hollow needle into the lesion and obtaining several cylindrical cores of tissue. If the mass is superficial and easily palpable core biopsies can easily be obtained by the surgeon and radiology guidance or localization to find the tumor may not be necessary. However, if the tumor is deep or small in size or only suspicious calcifications are noted by mammography, the surgeon may request a radiology to localize the tumor. This is usually done by using ultrasound to find the area of suspicion. After the area is found, it is snagged with a thin needle guide-wire which is inserted in the tumor or area of suspicion. Blue dye is then injected into the area so that it can be apparent to the surgeon where the tumor or suspicious area is located so the tumor or area of suspicion can be excised.

An alternative method to obtain biopsies or samplings of the tumor that is too deep or small for the surgeon to locate by hand is stereotactic needle biopsy. This procedure is less invasive. Instead of a surgical procedure a needle may be inserted into the suspicious area by directly using radiology imaging. Several needle cores of tissue can be obtained for evaluation. This procedure does not necessarily remove the entire lesion or mass.

If the biopsies of the mass or area of suspicion have been found to be malignant, the decisions that are made for your care should be based upon shared decision making between you and your physician. Enough information should be given to the you to make a decision based on current treatment regarding surgery, chemotherapy and radiation therapy.[8] Shared decision making makes you an active participant in the decision making process. You should expect your physician to spend more time with you if you have severe disease or cancer. Your quality of life is important. Once the diagnosis of cancer is made your physician will determine the stage or extent of the disease by using the results of the clinical examination, the surgical pathology report, CT or PET scan, liver and bone scan, chest X-ray and other tests that your physician may order. Make sure that you know and understand the results of your reports. Have copies of these reports made for you files. Go over the results with a family member or your personal health advocate. Do not be kept out of the loop when it concerns your treatment. Be a part of the decision making process.

I cannot stress enough that you should know your options in regards to surgical treatment. Eighteen states in the United States currently have legislation where the surgeon is required to give the patient information about available treatment options and the risks and benefits of the treatment options. A study conducted by Hawley at University of Michigan showed that more than half of breast cancer patients were ill informed about the risks and benefits of treatment options and over half did not know that the five year survival was similar for patients electing mastectomy (surgical breast removal) and those electing BCS (breast conserving surgery). [9]   If you are a patient contemplating surgery or a medical procedure, it is imperative that you take an active role in your treatment. Do not be a bystander in the process of your treatment, be an active participant. The authorization that you as a patient make for treatment is usually voluntarily given, but it is your duty be informed in order to give that consent. You must make sure that complete information has been given to you about the treatment and hold your physician accountable for disclosing that information. You have the right to the self-determination of your treatment and as I stated before some states have passed legislation to ensure that right of self-determination.

You need to know the nature of the treatment that you will receive. It should be explained to you about what the risks of the treatment are and what the benefits are. You should ask you physician if there are alternative approaches and treatments and ask what they are. Make sure that your physician explains to you the differences between conservative surgical treatments for breast cancer versus a mastectomy.

If it is too much for you to remember, take a friend or spouse with you to the office visit to help you ask questions. You should have a good patient-physician relationship. You should not be anxious in discussing treatment issues and fears when it concerns your health. You have the right to be concerned about losing a breast. You have the right to be afraid about dying. Let your physician know your concerns and fears.

References:

1. Evans, P.; J Am Coll Radiol. 2010;7:18-27.
2. Barclay, Laurie and Vega, C. Digital vs. Film Mammography Screening for Breast Cancer May Have Advantages, Medscape-WedMD, Sept.20, 2005. (NEJM, Sept.2005)
3. Plevritis, Sylvia K. et al., Breast MRI Screening Cost-Effective for BRCA1/2 Carriers at selected Ages. JAMA 2006; 295:2374-2384.
4. Zhu Q, et al "Early-stage invasive breast cancers: Potential role of optical tomography with US localization in assisting diagnosis" *Radiology* 2010; DOI: 10.1148/radiol.10091237.
5. Scott Lind, D. and Smith, BL, ASC Surgery Online. 2002; @WedMD, Inc.
6. Silverstein, Melvin J., International Consensus Conference Panel, Guideline Update, Journal of the American College of Surgeons, Oct. 12, 2005.
7. Mayo Clinic Health Information. MayoClinic.com, May 2006.
8. Moumjid, Nora, Carr and Egrave, Clinical issues in shared decision making applied to breast cancer, Health Expect 2003, Sept6(3):222-7.
9. Hawley ST, et al "Racial/ethnic disparities in knowledge about risks and benefits of breast cancer treatment: Does it matter where you go?" Health Serv Res 2008; 43: 1366-1387.
10. Malone, KE, et al. "Population-based study of the risk of secondary primary contralateral breast cancer associated with carrying a mutation on BRCA1 or BRCA2". J Clin Oncol 2010: DOI:10L 1200/JCO. 2009.24.2495.

Lessons To Be Learned

1) Screening mammography is still recommended for breast cancer screening and is the most important test a woman can undergo to reduce her chances of dying.
2) Breast cancer can occur in men. 1% of all breast cancers occur in men.
3) Women who are at average risk for breast cancer should start mammography screening at age 40 and follow-up exams as

recommended by their physician.

4) Women who are at high risk for breast cancer should have annual mammography and MRI at age 30.

5) Make sure that you keep track of the results of your mammogram and understand the results of your reports.

6) If you have changes in your breast do not delay contacting your physician.

7) If you have a breast mass or abnormal mammogram, do not postpone any additional tests that you physician may request.

8) If you have a breast mass do not delay getting a biopsy of the mass. Do not delay getting the diagnosis of a breast mass.

Benign Conditions of the Breast

- **Juvenile hypertrophy** also called macromastia is condition of the breast usually occurring post-puberty females where one or both breasts are enlarged and may require reduction in size of the breast by surgery.
- **Comedomastitis** is an inflammatory condition of the breast affecting the ducts
- **Lymphocytic mastitis** is an inflammatory condition of the breast usually associated with diabetes. It affects the lobules of the breast and is associates with a fibrosis and lymphocytes (a type inflammatory white blood cell).
- **Plasma cell mastitis** is an inflammatory condition of the breast where there is a preponderance of white cells called plasma cells that make up the inflammation.
- **Granulomatous mastitis** is an inflammatory condition of the breast lobules usually presenting in young women with recent pregnancy. It is usually bilateral (occurring in both breasts) and may develop small abscesses (accumulation of pus and pus tracts).
- **Giant cell arteritis** is a inflammatory condition of the medium size blood vessels of the breast and usually develops in postmenopausal women. Cells with giant nuclei may be a part of the inflammation.
- **Traumatic fat necrosis** is degeneration of the fat cells or adipose tissue of the breast secondary to trauma or blunt injury.
- **Fibrocystic change** is a condition of the female breast, a benign or non-cancerous process consisting of proliferative changes of ducts (adenosis or an increase of breast ducts), hyperplasia (increase of cells in breast ducts) and fibrosis (increase in supporting tissue of the breast) together with non-proliferative changes which may consist of distention or dilation of breasts ducts with the formation of cysts which may be small or large in size.
- **Apocrine metaplasia** a benign change in the cells lining the breast ducts in which they resemble cells lining apocrine glands or a modified sweat glands. These cells have abundant eosinophilic or highly pink cytoplasm.
- **Adenosis** is hyperplasia or increase of breast ducts or glands.
- **Sclerosing adenosis** is hyperplasia or increase of breast ducts or glands

associated with increased fibrosis of the breast stroma or supporting tissue.

- **Nodular adenosis** is an early form of sclerosing adenosis.

- **Ductal hyperplasia** is an increase of ducts or cells lining the ducts.

- **Intraductal papillomatosis** is a proliferative lesion in the breast duct in which there are increased papillary tufts or aggregates of cells with irregularly shaped bridges which extend into the lumen or opening of a breast duct.

- **Intraductal Papilloma** is a benign papillary tumor within a breast duct occurring at about 48 years of age. It occurs in large ducts of the nipple and may be associated with a bloody discharge from the nipple.

- **Adenomyoepithelioma** is a benign tumor-like adenosis, increase ducts or adenoma (benign tumor of glands or ducts) usually occurring in postmenopausal women.

- **Fibroadenoma** is the most common benign tumor of the breast occurring in the second and third decades of life. It is usually well circumscribed with well defined borders rounded borders. It has increased fibrous stroma or supporting tissue. The breast ducts or glands are compressed by the fibrous stroma.

- **Ductal adenoma** is a benign breast lump, well circumscribed with rounded borders arising from the wall of a duct or gland. It consists of the epithelial cells lining the duct and small cells called myoepithelial cells located between the duct cells. The tumor is composed of compressed tubules or ducts.

- **Benign phylloides tumor** resembles fibroadenoma with benign glands and fibrous stroma, except the stroma is slightly more cellular. This tumor after surgical removal has a recurrence of 50%.

Borderline Lesions and Intraductal Neoplasia

-**Atypical ductal hyperplasia** consists of changes in the cells of the ducts which are suggestive of a low grade carcinoma. The lesion has a 3 to 5 times increase risk for carcinoma.

-**Atypical lobular hyperplasia** consists of changes of the epithelial cells of the lobular ducts that resemble lobular carcinoma in situ but do not completely fill the majority of ducts. The lesion has a 4 to 5 times risk of developing breast cancer.

-**Borderline phylloides tumor** looks similar to phylloides tumor but the stroma has a moderate increase of cells under the microscope. There may be up to 5 cells with mitotic figures (cells actively dividing) noted per 10 microscopic high power fields. The borders of the tumor are irregular and extend into the adjacent normal breast tissue.

- **Ductal intraepithelial neoplasia or Ductal carcinoma in situ (DCIS)** is tumor confined to the cells lining the ducts. It spreads along the length of the breast ducts but does not invade the basement membrane or bottom of the breast ducts, nor extend into the breast tissue surrounding the ducts. The different patterns of DCIS are: cribiform, comedo, hypersecretory, papillary, micropapillary, neuroendocrine, secretory, signet ring cell, and solid. DCIS is associated with an 8 to 10 times risk for the development of breast cancer. The tumors are graded as grade 1 (low-grade), grade 2 (intermediate-grade) or grade 3 (high-grade).

World Health Organization Classification:
 Ductal intraepithelial neoplasia (DIN)

    DIN 1A, 1B, 1C, (DCIS grade 1 or low-grade)
    (epithelial atypia, atypical ductal hyperplasia)
    DIN 2 (DCIS grade 2 or intermediate-grade)
    DIN 3 (DCIS grade 3 or high-grade).

- **Lobular intraepithelial neoplasia (LIN3) or Lobular carcinoma in situ (LCIS)** usually occurs in the lobular ducts. The peak occurrence is in females in their fifties. It is usually not associated with microcalcifications and is found incidentally on examination. Approximately 75% of cases show involvement in multiple areas of the breast. The risk for the occurrence of invasive breast carcinoma or cancer is 30% and the risk of disease in both breasts is up to 20%.

- **Paget's Disease** is an weeping rash of the skin of the breast, usually of the nipple. It is type of carcinoma in situ of the skin of the breast that extends into the underlying breast ducts. 50% of such skin lesions of the breast may be associated with an underlying DCIS or invasive breast cancer.

Table 17.1

DCIS AND LCIS				
TYPE	**AGE**	**SIZE**	**TREATMENT**	**PROGNOSIS**
DCIS	<45 y/o	< .5cm	Lumpectomy alone	40%
		> .5 cm with + margins	-Lumpectomy alone or	40%
Comedo(67%)			-Lumpectomy, no node biopsy + radiation whole breast or	40%
Micropapillary				Usually Low Grade Invasive
Papillary(<2%)				
Hypersecretory-r				
Apocrine	54-56 y/o		-Mastectomy + s.node biopsy + Reconstruction	20% Invasive component
Cribiform(10%)				Usually Low Grade
Neuroendocrine	> 60 y/o		———	Usually Low Grade
LCIS	53 y/o		Watching +/or Ipsilateral or bilateral mastectomy	Minimal risk dying, 5% invasive, 25% risk of invasion
PAGET'S DISEASE (CIS OF SKIN)			Excision + radiation or radiation alone	50% with DCIS or Invasive Tumor

Malignant Neoplasms of Breast

- **Invasive ductal carcinoma, NOS** (not otherwise specified) is the most common malignant tumor of the terminal breast ducts which invades the and extends into the surrounding breast tissue. The tumor is arranged usually in cords and sheets of cells that may extend into breast lymphatics channels and blood vessels.
- **Cribiform carcinoma** is a low-grade invasive carcinoma with a cribiform (cart-wheel) pattern.
- **Invasive lobular carcinoma** is malignant tumor of the lobular ducts. The cells of the duct invade and extend into the surrounding breast tissue. Classically, the cells are of small size, low nuclear grade and may have a small lumen (round opening) in the cytoplasm that contains mucin. The tumor has a characteristic "Indian file" pattern. The different patterns or variants of lobular carcinoma are: solid, trabecular, signet ring, histiocytoid, pleomorphic and alveolar.
- **Tubulolobular carcinoma** (mixed ductal and lobular carcinoma) is rare. It consists of typical invasive lobular carcinoma mixed with angular shaped ducts or tubules. The average age of occurrence is 60 years. About 30% of the tumors are multifocal (occur in multiple areas) of the breast. The tumor usually occurs in only one breast. Metastases (spread of the cancer to lymph nodes and other sites) occurs in about 30% of cases.
- **Mucinous (colloid) carcinoma** is a carcinoma of the breast that appears gelatinous. It is a low grade or well differentiated cancer with a 5 year survival of over 90%. It usually occurs in elderly women.
- **Clear Cell (Glycogen-Rich) carcinoma** is a rare breast carcinoma, less than 3% of breast carcinomas. The prognosis is similar to other breast cancers. The cells may have eosinophilic (deep pink) or clear cytoplasm and usually contain glycogen (complex starch).
- **Inflammatory carcinoma** is an aggressive breast cancer. The skin of the breast clinically has a peau d'orange(orange peal) appearance which indicates extensive involvement of the lymphatic vessels or channels.
- **Juvenile carcinoma (Secretory carcinoma)** is a rare carcinoma of the breast occurring usually in children and has a 5 year 100% survival.
- **Medullary carcinoma** is less than 1% of breast cancers and usually

occurs in women less than 50 years old. It is common in Japanese women and is associated with the breast cancer antigen BRCA1. The cancer has large cells. The borders of the tumor are pushing and there is a prominent inflammation consisting of lymphocytes. The prognosis of this cancer is better than invasive ductal carcinoma and most breast cancers.

- **Adenoid cystic carcinoma** is very rare, less than 1% of breast cancers. It occurs in women predominantly ages 50 to 60 years. It has a very good prognosis and spread of the tumor outside the breast and recurrence is rare.

- **Apocrine carcinoma** is a rare breast carcinoma, less than 4% of breast cancers. It usually occurs in women in their forties. The cells have deep eosinophilic (pink) cytoplasm and an eccentric (off to the side) nucleus. Hormone receptors, ER and PR are usually negative.

- **Metaplastic carcinoma** (spindle cell or sarcomatoid carcinoma, or carcinosarcoma (combined sarcoma with carcinoma)) occurs in less than 5% of breast cancers and is usually more aggressive than invasive ductal carcinoma.

- **Neuroendocrine carcinoma** is a breast cancer which features rosettes, and small cells with rare mitoses (cells in division). It is 5% of breast cancers.

- **Oncocytic carcinoma** consists of cells will granular eosinophilic (pink) cytoplasm with a low nuclear grade.

-**Lipid rich carcinoma** is less than 2% of breast malignancies and has a very poor prognosis.

-**Tubular carcinoma** is less than 6% of breast tumors and consists of very well differentiated ducts or tubules. It occurs in women at the average age of 50 years and may involve multiple sites of the breast in about 30% of cases and bilateral (occur in both breasts) in 40% of cases. There is a family history of breast cancer in about 40% of cases. The prognosis is good clinically even when the cancer has spread to axillary (under the arm) lymph nodes.

-**Malignant lymphoma** is less than 1% of breast malignancies. The tumor is a primary lymphoma a tumor of malignant lymphocytes in the breast. If the lymphoma is confined to the breast and has no association of lymphomatous disease outside the breast at the time of diagnosis it is a primary lymphoma. Secondary breast lymphoma is also rare. It is usually associated with evidence of a previous existing low-grade lymphoma not arising in the breast but secondarily involves the breast.

-Metastatic carcinoma is cancer which has spread to other organs or lymph nodes from a site other than the original tumor site. Breast cancers usually spread or metastasize to lymph nodes, liver, lung, bone and brain. There are cancers that may spread or metastasize to the breast. The most common are serous carcinoma of the ovary and the peritoneum (cell lining of the abdominal cavity), carcinoid tumors of the intestines, mucoepidermoid carcinoma, small cell (oat cell) carcinoma, squamous cell carcinoma of the lung, malignant melanoma, colon cancer and a rare childhood tumors, and rhabdomyosarcoma.

- **Plasmacytoma,** a tumor of plasma cells is rare. Most cases are from Multiple Myeloma, a systemic malignancy of plasma cells in the blood and may occur years after a patient has been treated and in remission.

- **Amyloid tumors** are rare and may occur in elderly women with Multiple Myeloma. The tumor is composed of the accumulation of amyloid, a type AA protein.

- **Myeloid sarcoma or granulocytic sarcoma or chloroma** is a neoplasm of white or myeloid blood cells, namely myeloblasts or immature white blood cells, and is associated with myeloid leukemia.

- **Malignant phylloides tumo**r is very rare and is aggressive in up to 25% of cases. It can metastasize or spread to the lung, bone and brain. Other types of stromal cells or supporting cells other than fibroblasts may be present namely, rhabdomyosarcoma (sarcoma of muscle cells), liposarcoma (sarcoma of fat cells) or osteosarcoma(sarcoma of bone). When these cells are present they indicate poor prognosis.

- **Sarcomas** of breast may be low grade or high grade depending upon the nuclear grade and the amount of cells appearing in mitotic phase (cell division per high power field) when examined under the microscope. High grade tumors have more mitoses and are associated with death from metastases in 30% of cases. **Angiosarcoma, lymphangiosarcoma and malignant hemagioendothelioma** are tumors of vascular channels usually in young women and in older women. These tumors are associated with post radiation therapy. **Leiomyosarcoma** is a tumor of spindle shaped smooth muscle cells. **Liposarcoma** is less than 0.3% of breast sarcomas, consisting of malignant fat cells or lipocytes. The median age of occurrence is 47 years. The tumor may be aggressive if occurring during pregnancy. Prognosis is poor with death occurring within 18 months.

-Myofibrosarcoma is a tumor of myofibroblasts and extremely rare.

-Osteosarcoma is a tumor of bone modeling cells (osteoblasts, osteoclasts) and fibroblasts. Malignant osteoid or bone matrix is present.

-Rhabdomyosarcoma is a tumor of primitive skeletal muscle cells or rhabdomyoblasts. The cells may have cross striations as seen in skeletal muscle fibers.

-Stromal sarcoma is a sarcoma of the stromal or supporting cells surrounding benign (non-cancerous) ducts or epithelium. It occurs in ages 30 to 90 years.

MALIGNANT TUMORS OF THE BREAST   Table 17.2

TUMOR	INCIDENCE	AGE	SIZE	TREATMENT	PROGNOSIS
Ductal NOS	75-80%			Surgery < 1 cm	5 yr 90%
Cribiform	0.3 - 3.5%	39 – 85 yrs	4.2 cm	> 1 cm Surgery + Radiation	
Comedo					
Colloid/Mucinous	3%				10 yr > 90%
Hypersecretory	Very rare				Usually low grade
Adenoid Cystic	<1%	25 – 80 yrs	1 – 3 cm	Excision	Good
Adenosquamous			1 – 9 cm		May recur locally
Apocrine	0.3 - 14 %	34 – 78 yrs	.5 – 5 cm		5 yr 90%
Glycogen-Rich	1 - 3%	60 yrs			5 yr 90%
Inflammatory	1 - 2%	24 – 62 yrs		Pre-op radiation+ Chemotherapy + Mastectomy	15 yr 45% responders to induction Rx
Lipid Rich	1.4- 1.6%	33 - 81 yrs	1 -15 cm		1 yr 62%
Medullary	< 1%	< 50 yrs			> 5 yr 90%
Metaplastic	< 5%		1 – 21 cm	Excision/ Mastectomy	< 5 yr 90%
Micropapillary	< 2%	25 – 92 yrs	.1 – 10 cm		Poor
Mucinous	1 -6%	35 – 75 yrs			
Cystadeno carcinoma	Very Rare	49 – 96 yrs	1 – 19 cm		
Lobular	0.7 - 15%	26 - 86 yrs	Poorly defined masses		
Mucoepidermoid	Rare				
Myoepithelial	Rare				
Signet Ring Cell	2 - 4%	33 – 87 yrs			Poor Aggressive

Secretory	Rare	3- 87 yrs	6 - 12 cm	Excision / mastectomy	Age dependent
Neuroendocrine	5%				5 yr 90%
Oncocytic	Rare				
Papillary	1 - 2%	63 – 67 yrs			>5 yr 90%
Juvenile (secretory)	Rare	Children			5 yr 100%
Small cell	Rare	43 – 70 yrs	1 – 5 cm		
Squamous cell	Very Rare		2 - 12 cm		
Tubular	0.4 –8%	50 yrs	1 cm		Very Good
Tubulolobular	Rare	43 – 79 yrs	.5 – 2.5 cm		Intermediate
Sarcoma-NOS	<1%				
Low Grade					Good
High Grade	<.05%	Young +/or 5 - 10 yrs post radiation		Complete Excison	Poor
Angiosarcoma					
Low Grade/ High Grade	Rare			Excison + Chemo	Better Poor
Leiomyosarcoma	Rare	50 yrs	1 - 5 cm	Wide Excision	Poor
Liposarcoma	Rare	19 – 76 yrs	8 - 19cm		May be aggressive
Myofibrosarcoma	Rare	27 – 89 yrs			Poor
Osteosarcoma	Rare	27 – 89 yrs	4.5 - 6 cm	Wide Excision	5 yr 38%
Stromal sarcoma	Rare	Elderly	3 cm	Excision	
Amyloid tumor	1%	30 – 60 yrs			
Lymphoma	Not common	31 – 73 yrs			
Granulocytic sarcoma		21 – 56 yrs		Radiation + Chemo	Associated with AML

ATLAS

Slide 1   Subsegmental ducts

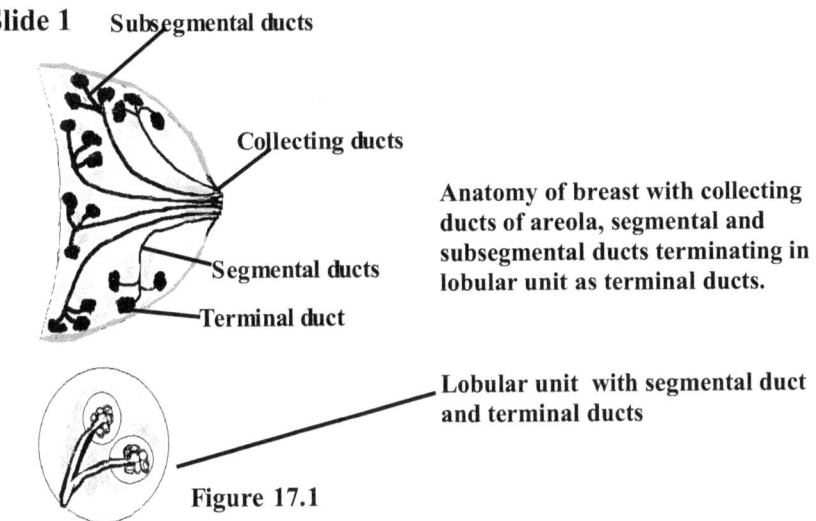

Collecting ducts

Anatomy of breast with collecting ducts of areola, segmental and subsegmental ducts terminating in lobular unit as terminal ducts.

Segmental ducts

Terminal duct

Lobular unit with segmental duct and terminal ducts

Figure 17.1

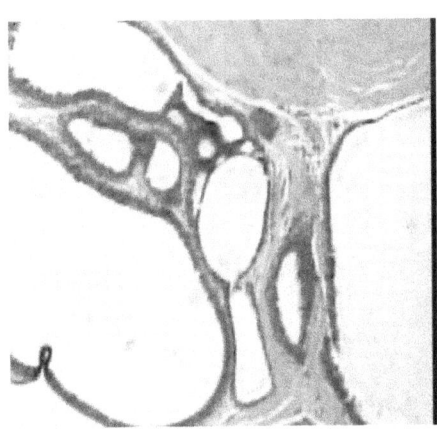

Figure 17.2. Dilated Breast ducts with cystic change

Figure17.3. Ducts with secretions.

Fat cells 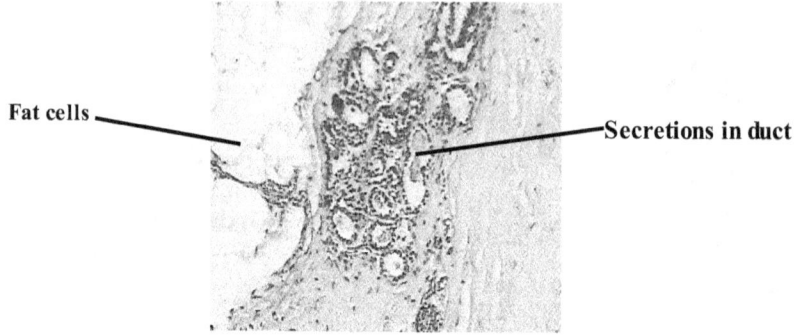 Secretions in duct

Figure 17.4. Adenosis

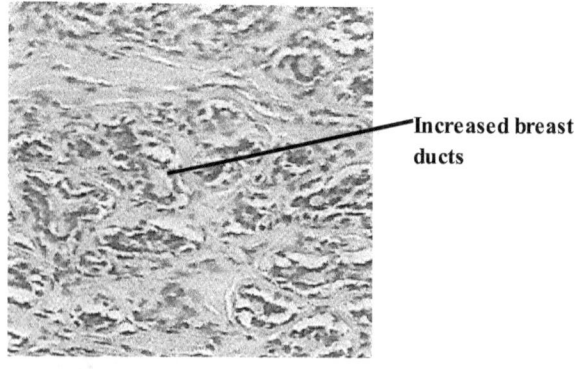 Increased breast ducts

Figure17.5. Increased fibrous tissue and ducts, adenosis

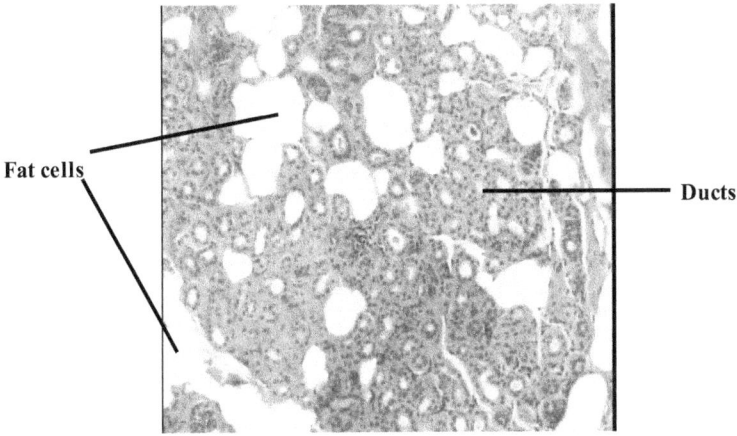

Fat cells

Ducts

Figure17.6. Increased fibrous tissue and ducts, fibrodenosis.

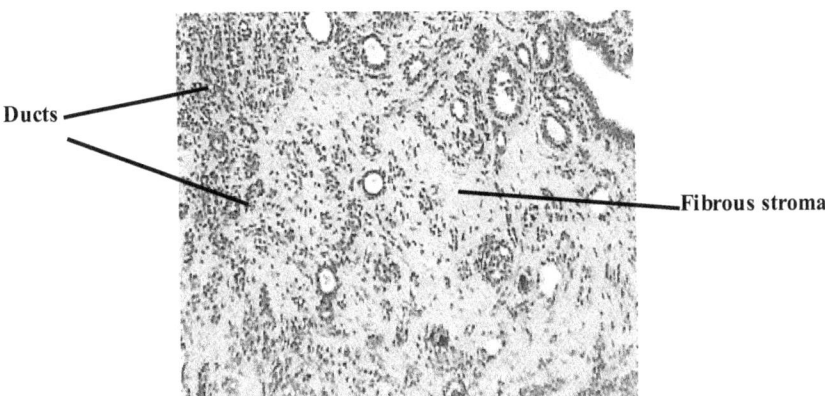

Ducts

Fibrous stroma

Figure17.7. Fibroadenosis with cystic change and microcalcification.

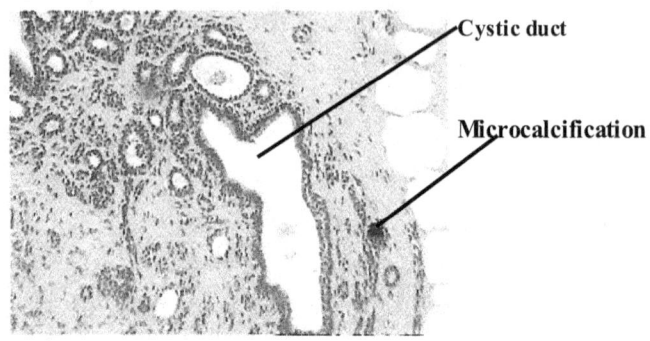

Cystic duct

Microcalcification

Figure17.8. Ducts with microcalcifications.

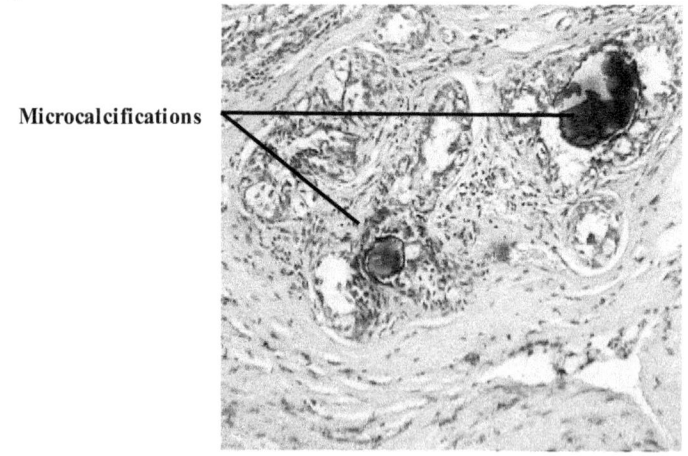

Microcalcifications

Figure 17.9. Duct with microcalcification.

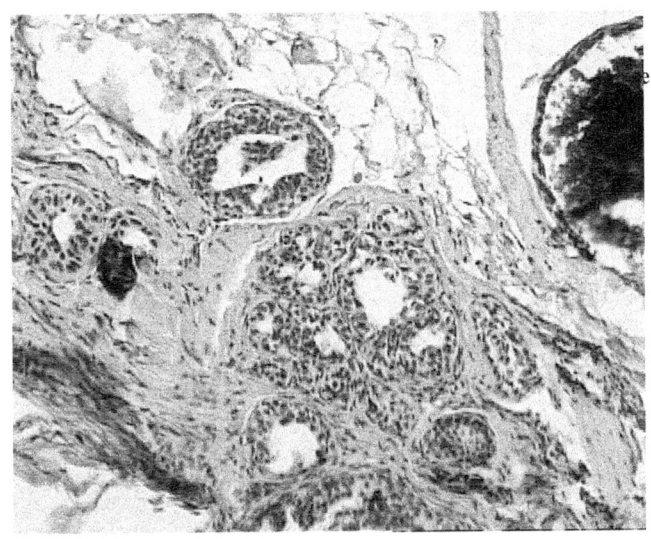

Figure 17.10. Lobular ducts with microcalcifications

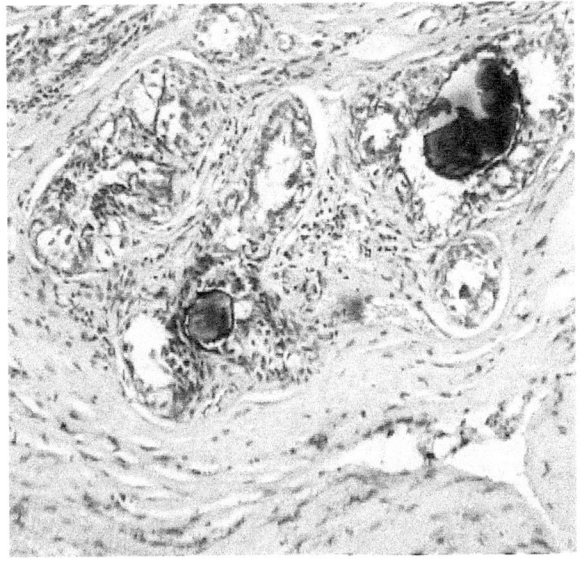

Figure 17.11.   Elongated segmented ducts

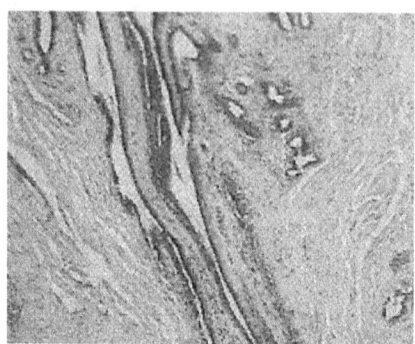

Figure 17.12.   Proliferative breast changes

Increased ducts

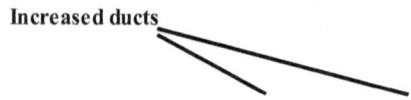

Figure 17.13.   Intraductal papillomatosis

Note small papillae
in duct

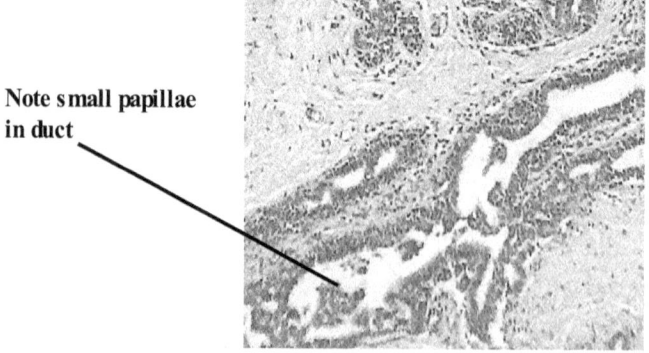

Figure 17.14. Proliferative breast with intraductal papillomatosis

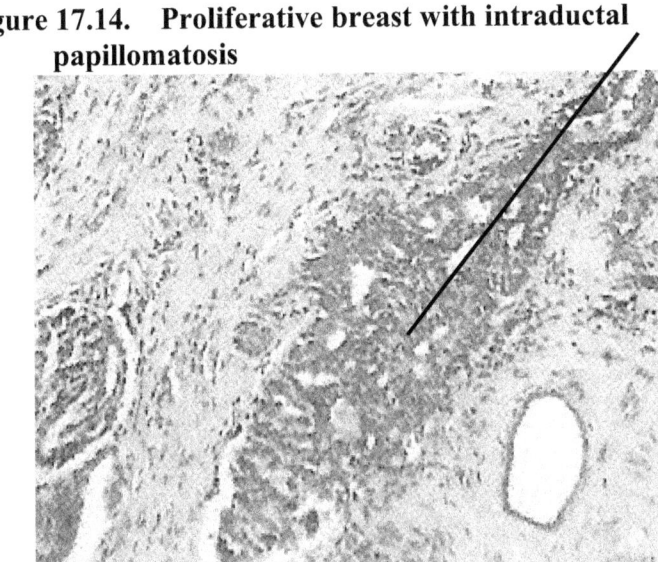

Figure 17.15. Proliferative breast with intraductal papillomatosis

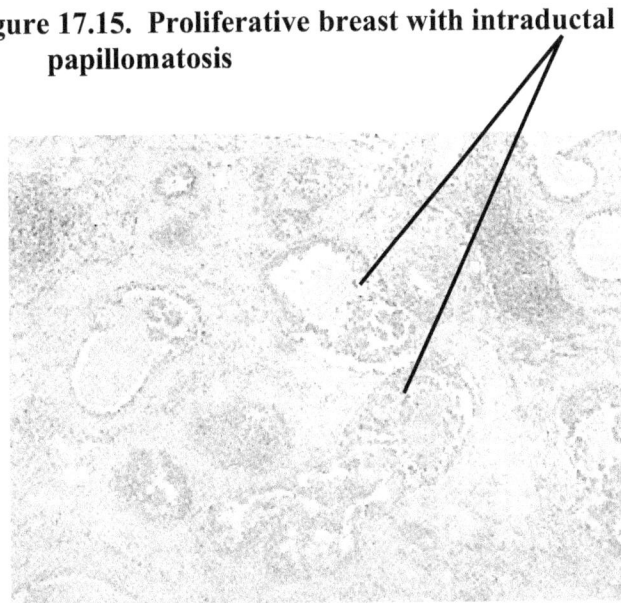

Figure 17.16.   Ductal hyperplasia

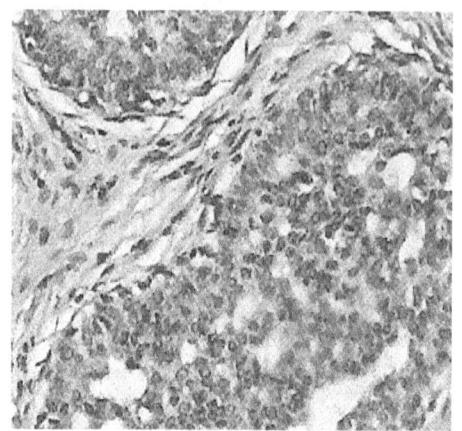

Figure 17.17.   Ductal hyperplasia

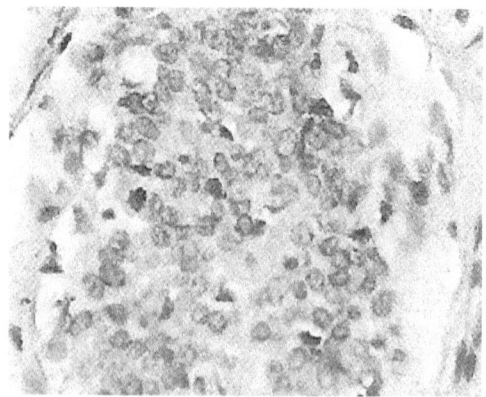

Figure 17.18. Lobular duct hyperplasia

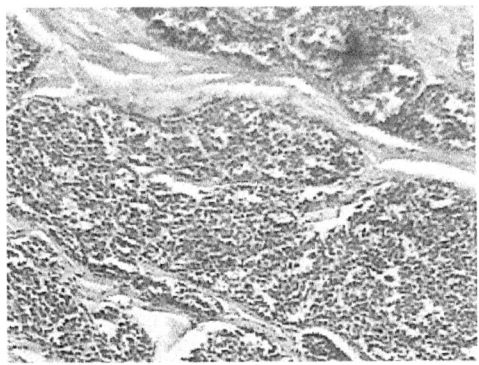

Note fullness of ducts

Figure 17.19. Lobular neoplasia

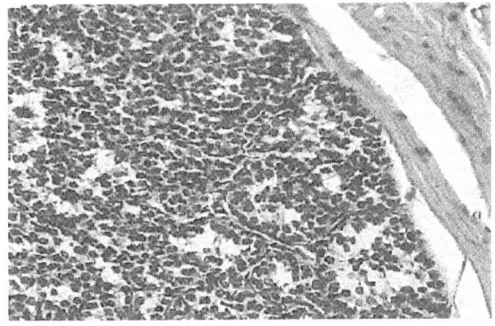

Figure 17.20. Lobular neoplasia

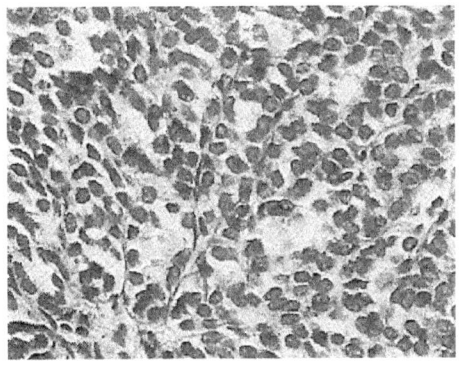

Figure 17.21.   Lobular neoplasia – carcinoma in situ

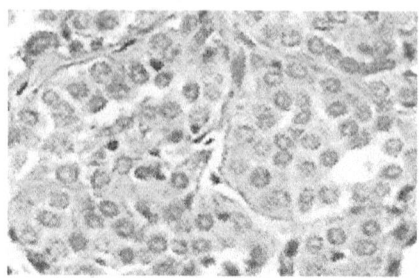

Figure 17.22.   Ductal hyperplasia

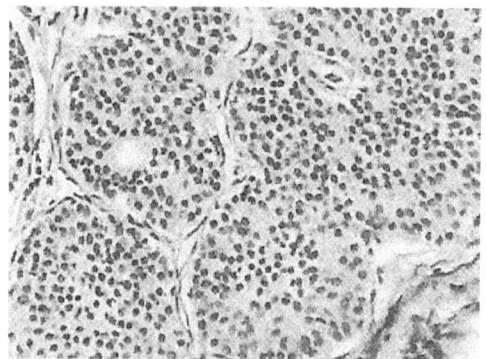

Figure 17.23. DCIS(carcinoma in situ) cribiform type

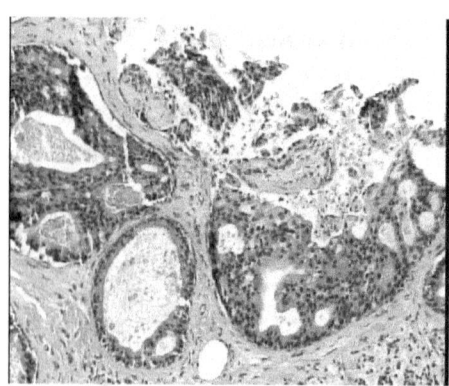

Figure 17.24. Ductal Carcinoma, comedo-type

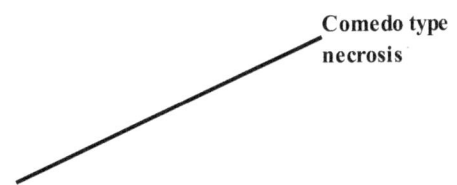

Comedo type
necrosis

Figure 17.25. Ductal carcinoma, cribiform type

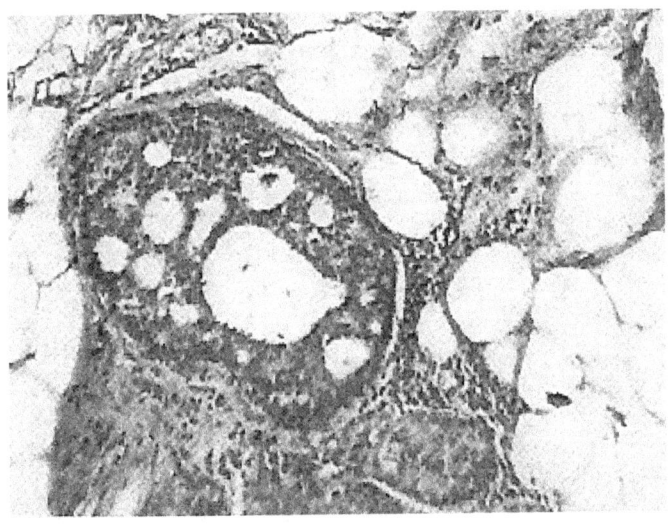

Figure 17.26. Ductal carcinoma, mixed cribiform and comedo type

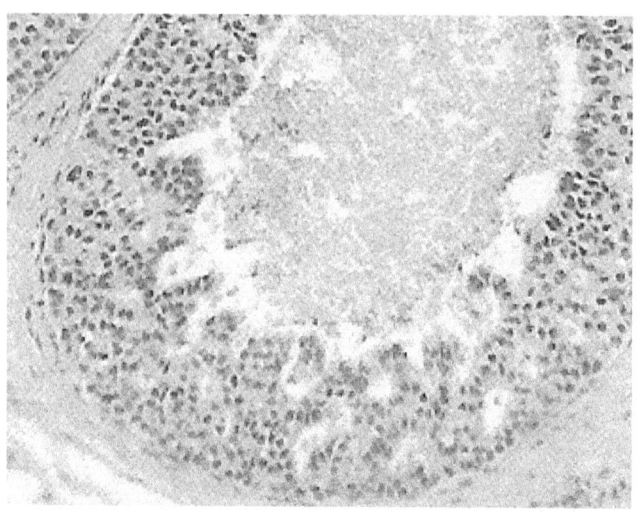

Figure 17.27. Invasive ductal carcinoma, comedo type with necrosis and microcalcifications

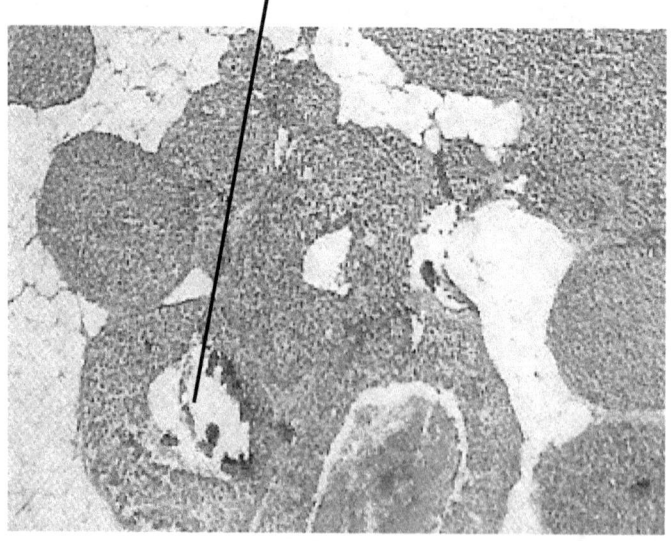

Figure 17.28. Mastectomy with left axillary lymph nodes attached

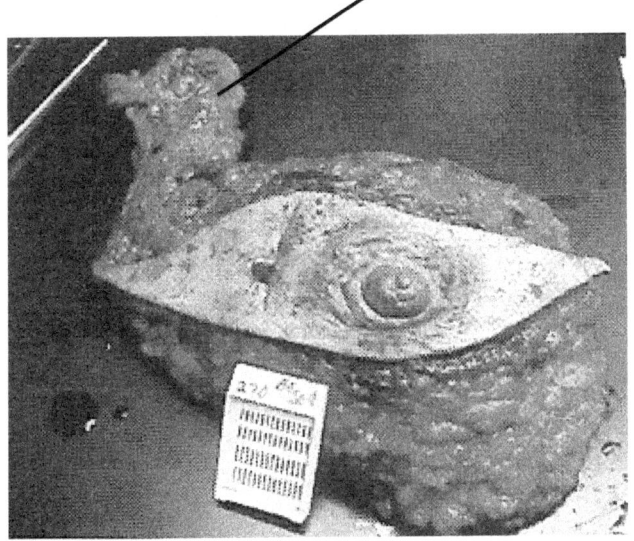

Figure 17.29. Mastectomy with axillary nodes attached left upper corner. Note scar to left of areola at previous biopsy site.

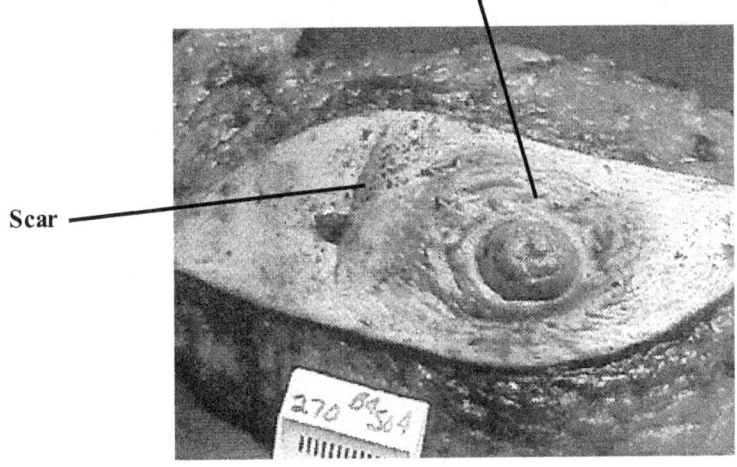

**Figure 17.30. Previous biopsy site with pink white
tumor and foci of hemorrhage.**

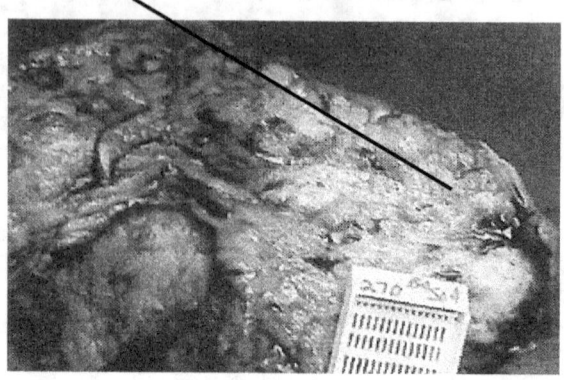

**Figure 17.31. Previous biopsy with hemorrhage and
tumor.**

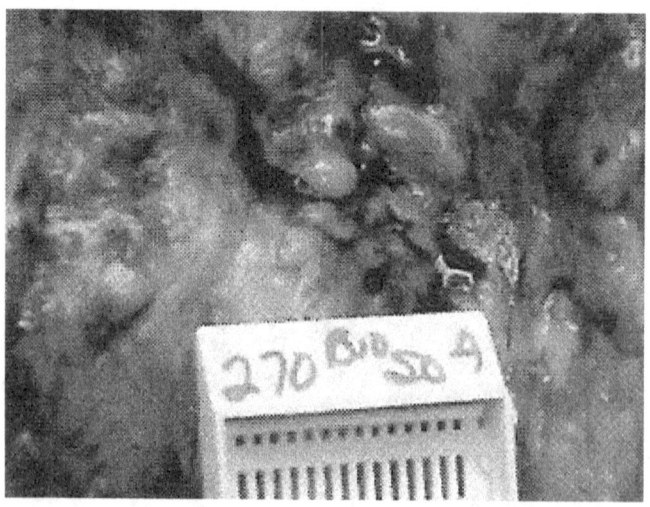

Figure 17.32. Closer view of tumor with hemorrhage

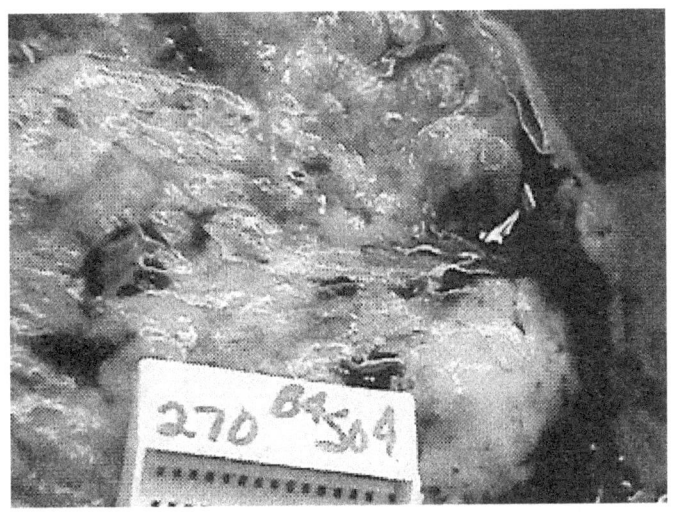

Figure 17.33. Invasive ductal carcinoma, NOS

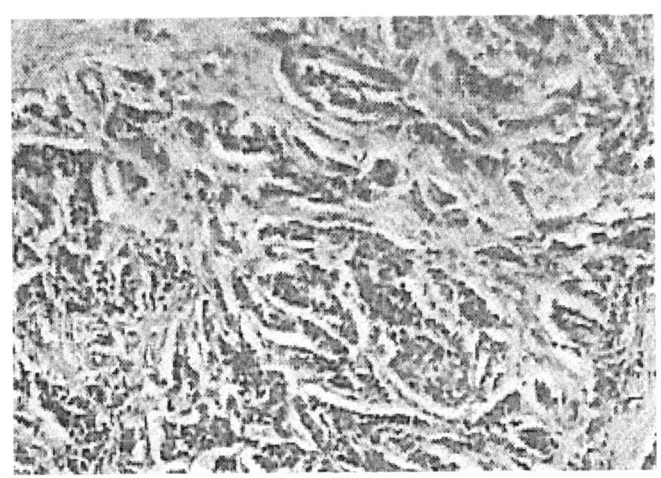

Figure 17.34. Invasive ductal carcinoma

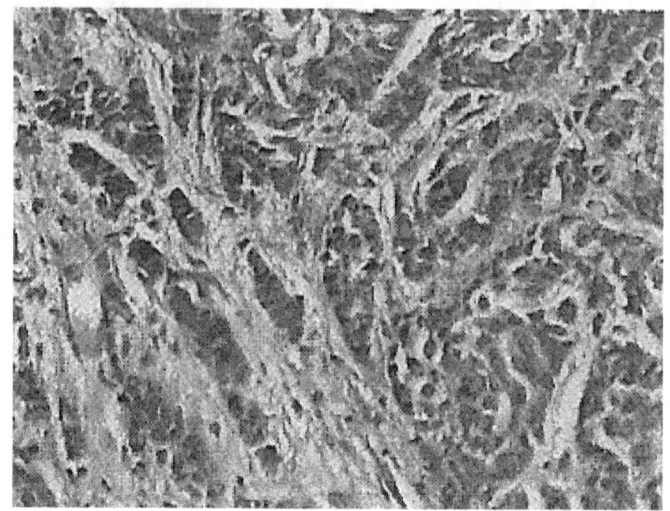

Figure 17.35. Invasive ductal carcinoma

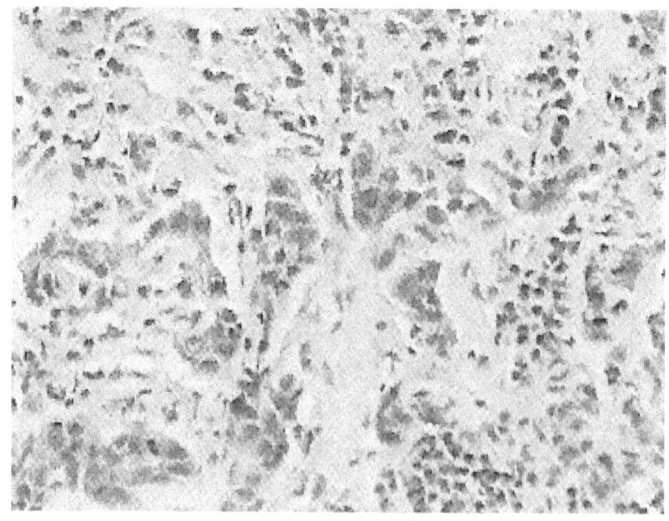

Figure 17.36. Invasive ductal carcinoma

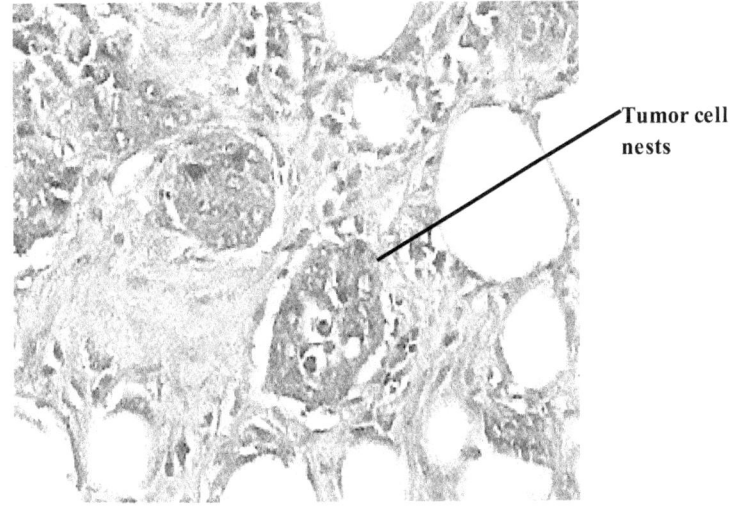

Tumor cell
nests

Figure 17.37. Grade 2. Invasive ductal carcinoma

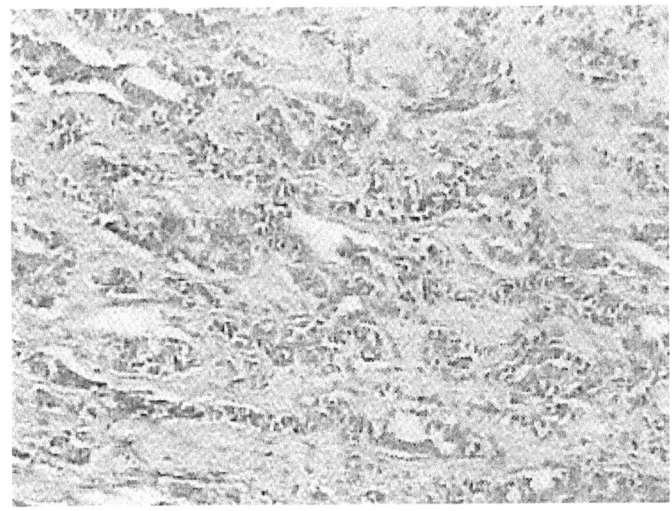

Figure 17.38.   Grade 3 invasive ductal carcinoma

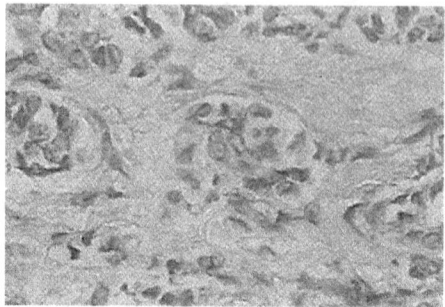

Figure 17.39.   Invasive ductal carcinoma

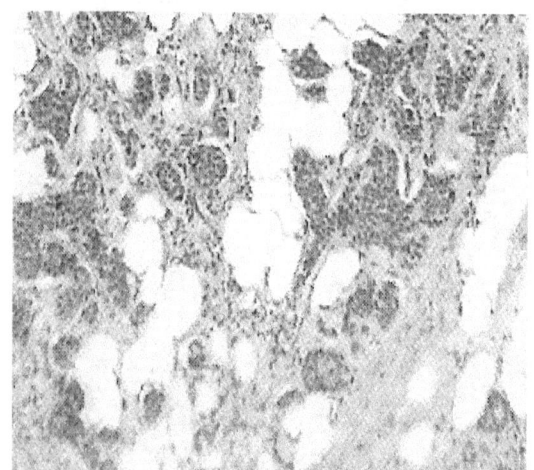

Figure 17.40. Metastatic ductal carcinoma, lymph node

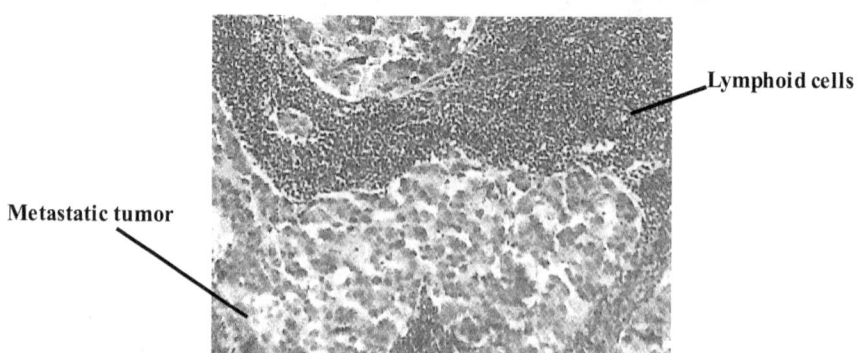

Figure 17.41. Invasive ductal carcinoma

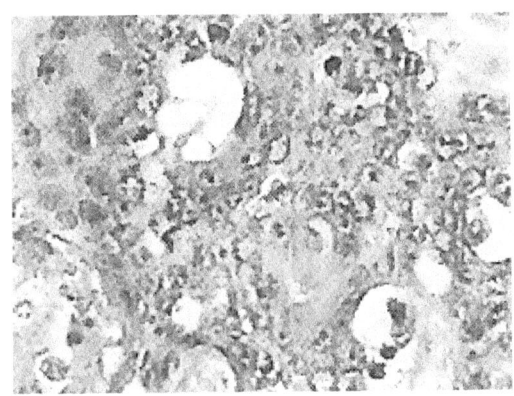

Figure 17.42. Grade 2 invasive ductal carcinoma

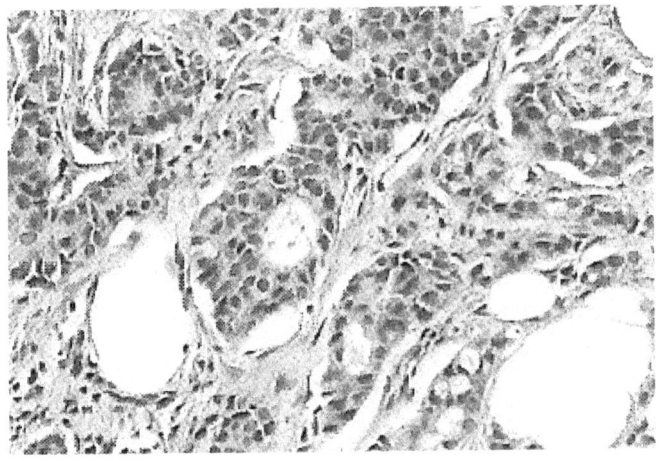

Figure 17.43.   Invasive ductal carcinoma

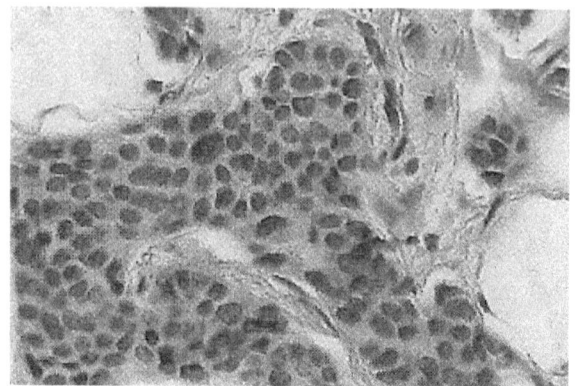

Figure 17.44. DCIS, Grade 1

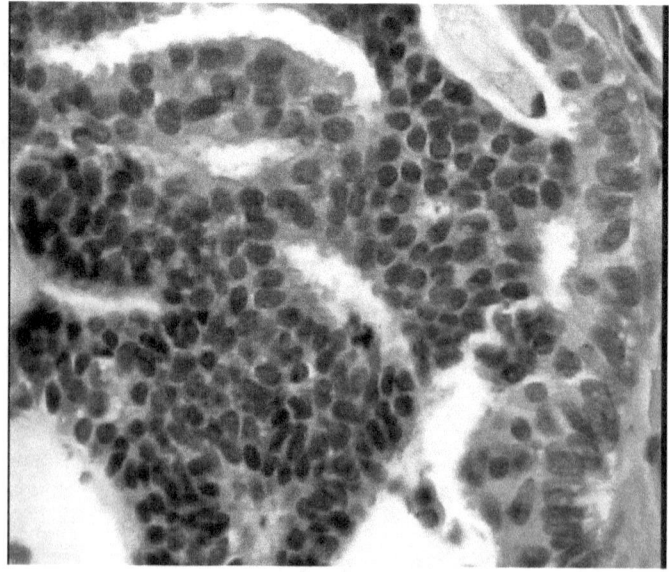

Figure 17.45. Invasive ductal carcinoma

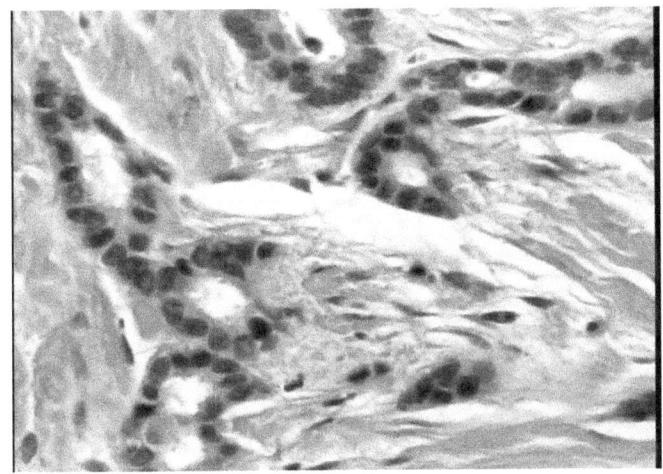

Figure 17.46. Grade 3 invasive ductal carcinoma

Note: high nuclear grade and no glands

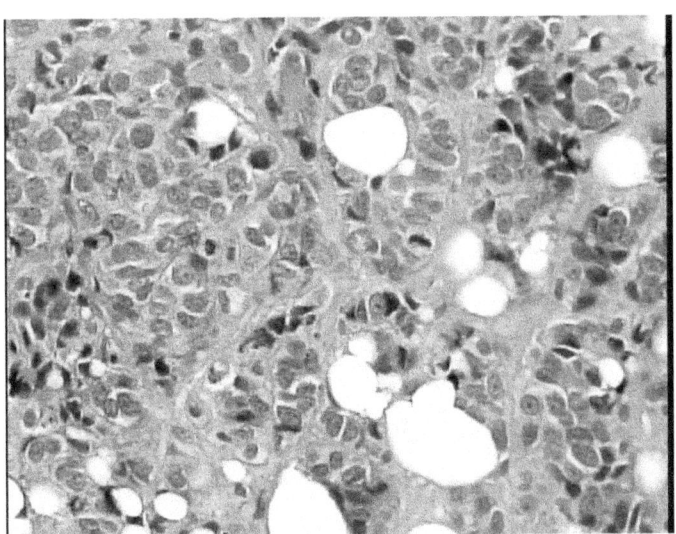

Figure 17.47. Tubular carcinoma

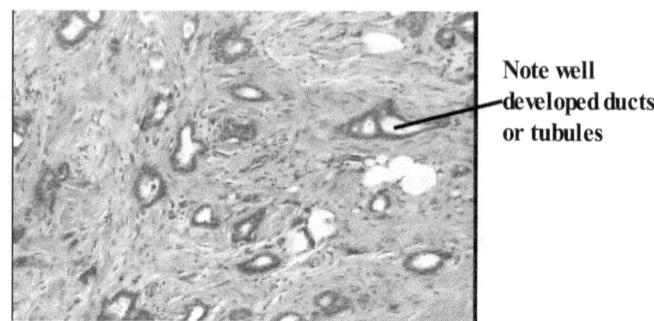

Note well
developed ducts
or tubules

Figure 17.48. Signet ring carcinoma

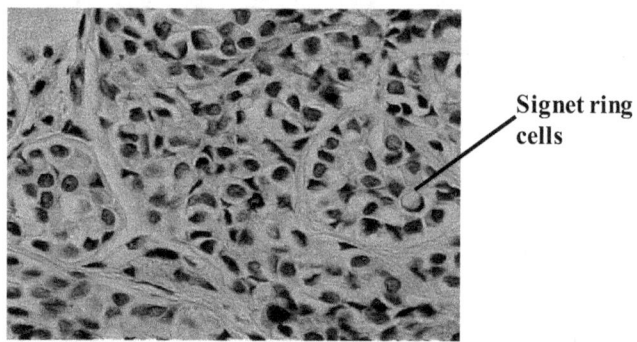

Signet ring
cells

Figure 17.49. Low grade sarcoma

Spindle shaped
cells

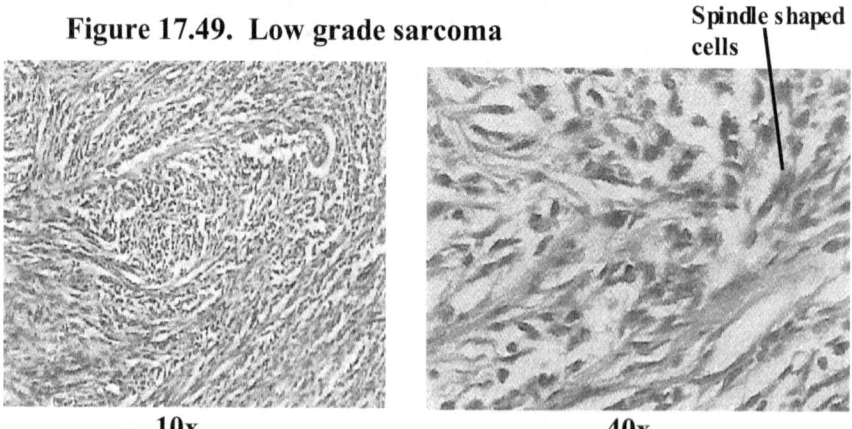

10x   40x

Figure 17.50. Estrogen receptor positive (ER+)

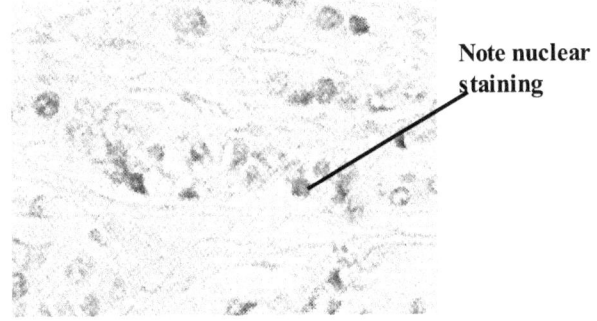

Note nuclear staining

Figure 17.51. Progesterone receptor positive (PR+)

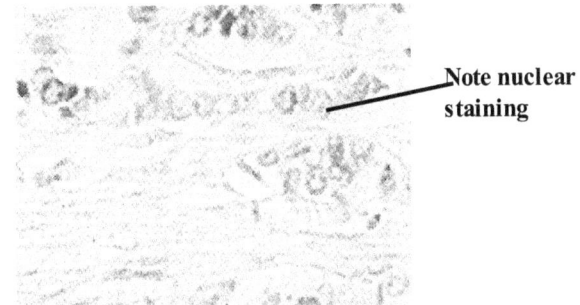

Note nuclear staining

Figure 17.52. Her2Neu receptor positive (Her2Neu+)

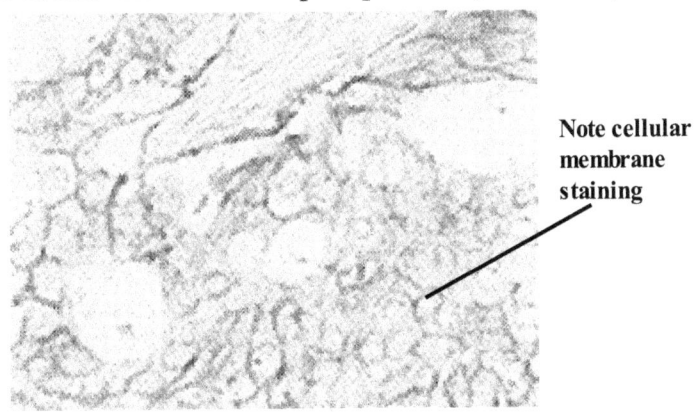

Note cellular membrane staining

Figure 17.53. Estrogen Receptor Positive (ER+)

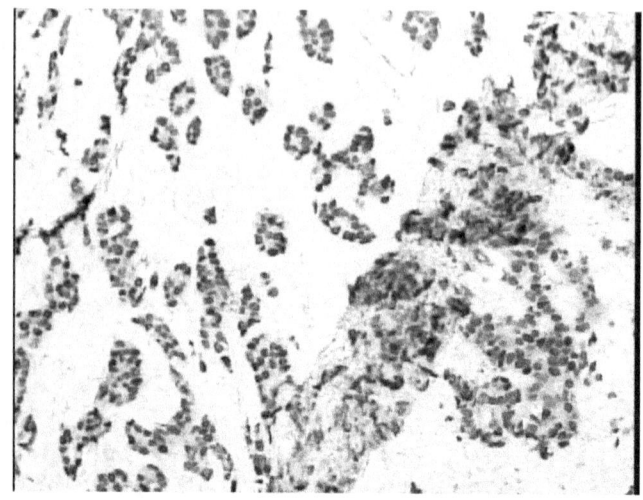

Figure 17.54. DCIS, Progesterone receptor positive (PR+)

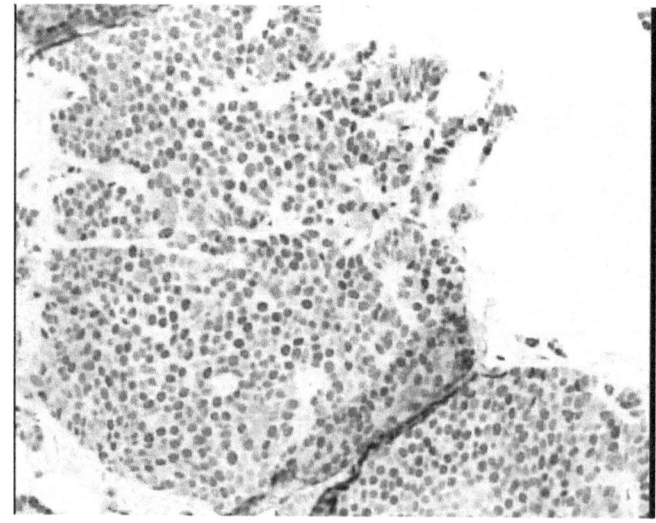

BREAST CANCER GRADING

A pathologist evaluates the tumor under the microscope and assesses the histological characteristics of the tumor to determine the histological grade of the breast tumor. The tumor grade is a prognostic indicator. There are two histologic grading systems commonly used, Scarff-Bloom-Richardson and the Elston/Nottingham system. Each uses a point grade scoring system for the following characteristics: tubule (t) formation, nuclear (n) grade and mitoses (m) .

Scarff-Bloom-Richardson Grading Schema

Tubule (or duct) formation (t) :
- \>75% of tumor consists of tubules= 1 point
- 10-75% of tumor consists of tubules= 2 points
- <10% of tumor consists of tubules= 3 points

Nuclear grade (n) (the amount of pleomorphism or variation in size or shape of the nucleus):
- Small uniform nuclei   = 1 point
- Moderate nuclear variation= 2 points
- Marked nuclear variation = 3 points

Mitoses (m) (number of mitotic figures observed when examining t0 microscopic high power fields using a 40x objective of the microscopic):
- 0-5   = 1 point
- 6-10 = 2 points
- \>11   = 3 points

The t, n, m points are added together to determine a total score and the differentiation of the tumor as follows:
- Well differentiated   (Grade I)   3-5 points
- Moderately differentiated (Grade II)   6-7 points
- Poorly differentiated   (Grade III) 8-9 points

BREAST CANCER STAGING

The stage of a tumor is the extent of spread of the tumor or cancer in the body. It is a predictor of survival and a prognostic index. The extent of disease and tumor spread can be determined clinical evaluation by physical examination, by radiologic tests like mammograms, X-rays, liver, brain, bone and CT and PET scans, biopsies, evaluation of the resected tumor. The clinical physical should include examination of the breast, the tumor size, mobility, associated skin changes if any and the presence or absence and mobility of lymph nodes, their involvement and evidence of the tumor spreading to distant sites or organs. The American Joint Committee for Cancer (AJCC) staging is used for both clinical and pathologic staging and classification of disease. It is based upon the evaluation of the primary tumor size (T), the spread of the cancer regional lymph nodes (N), and distant metastases (M), that is spread to lymph nodes other than axillary, internal mammary or pectoral lymph nodes and to other organs. The AJCC staging is as follows:

Primary Tumor (T)

Tx   primary tumor cannot be assessed (insufficient tissue to evaluate the highest T

T0   no evidence of primary tumor

Tis   carcinoma in situ (DCIS, LCIS or Paget's disease without an underlying invasive tumor)

T1   tumor size $\leq$ 2 cm

T1mic microinvasion $\leq$ 1 mm (.1 cm) (if multiple foci the size of the largest focus is used)

T1a   tumor size >1 mm to 5 mm (.1 cm to .5 cm)

T1b   tumor size 5 mm to 1cm (.5 cm to 1 cm)

T1c   tumor size 1 cm to 2 cm

T2   tumor size 2 cm to 5 cm

T3   tumor size $\geq$ than 5 cm

T4   tumor of any size with direct extension to chest wall or skin as noted below

T4a   extension to chest wall (ribs, intercostal muscles and serratus anterior muscle), excluding pectoralis muscle

T4b   edema (including peau d'orange) or ulceration of the skin

of the breast or satellite, non-connecting skin nodules
confined to the same breast

T4c   both T4a and T4b

T4d   inflammatory carcinoma (by clinical diagnosis)

Regional lymph nodes (N): (p-pathology assessment)

pNx   regional lymph nodes cannot be assessed for study (i.e.
        The lymph nodes may have been previously removed or
        not removed for study)

N0   No lymph nodes involved

pN0   no regional lymph nod metastasis or no additional
        examination for isolated tumor cells

pN(i+) no regional lymph node metastasis histologically, negative
        IHC.

pN(i-) no regional lymph node metastasis histologically, positive
        IHC, no IHC cluster greater than .2mm

pN(mol-) no regional lymph node metastasis histologically,
        negative molecular findings (RT-PCR)

pN(mol+) no regional lymph node metastasis histologically,
        positive molecular findings (RT-PCR)

N1   Involved lymph node or nodes

pN1   metastasis in 1-3 axillary lymph nodes or internal
        mammary nodes with microscopic disease detected by
        sentinel lymph node dissection but not clinically apparent

pN1mi micrometastasis (greater than .2mm, none greater than
        2mm)

pN1a   metastasis in 1-3 axillary lymph nodes

pN1b   metastasis in internal mammary nodes with microscopic
        disease detected by sentinel lymph node dissection but not
        clinically apparent

pN1c   metastasis in 1-3 axillary lymph nodes and in
        infraclavicular lymph nodes, or in clinically apparent
        ipsilateral internal mammary lymph nodes in the presence

of one or more positive axillary lymph nodes, or in more than 3 axillary lymph nodes with clinically negative microscopic metastasis in internal mammary lymph nodes, or in ipsilateral supraclavicular lymph nodes

N2 Involved lymph nodes fixed to one another
pN2a metastasis in 4-axillary lymph nodes, or in clinically

apparent internal mammary lymph nodes in the absence of axillary lymph node metastasis

pN2a metastasis in 4-axillary lymph nodes (at least one tumor deposit greater than 2 mm)

pN2b metastasis in clinically apparent internal mammary lymph nodes in the absence of axillary lymph node metastasis pN3a metastasis in 10+ axillarylymph nodes (at least one tumor deposit 2mm or more), or metastasis to infraclavicular lymph nodes

N3 Internal mammary nodes involved
pN3b metastasis in clinically apparent ipsilateral internal mammary lymph nodes in the presence of 1+ positive axillary lymph nodes, or in 4 or more axillary lymph nodes and in internal mammary lymph nodes with microscopic disease detected by sentinel lymph node dissection but not clinically apparent by imaging studies or clinically examination

Distant Metastasis (M)
Mx   distant metastasis cannot be assessed
M0   no distant metastasis
M1   distant metastasis (lung, liver, bone, etc)

Stage grouping

Stage 0	Tis N0 M0
Stage I	T1 N0 M0
Stage IIA	T0-T1 N1 M or T2 N0 M0
Stage IIB	T2 N1 M or T3 N0 M0
Stage IIIA	T1-T2 N2 M0 or T3 N1-N2 M0
Stage IIIB	T4 N0-N2 M0
Stage IIIC	Any T pN3 M0
Stage IV	Any T, Any N M1

Lessons To Be Learned

1) Familiarize yourself with the different types of breast cancer, tumor grading and tumor staging to equip yourself to be able to ask questions your physician about the grade and stage of your tumor.
2) Be prepared to ask you physician about the grading and staging of your tumor and your prognosis.
3) Ask your physician whether or not you need systemic chemotherapy and radiation therapy.
4) Make sure that the oncologist, radiation oncologist and the surgeon to whom you will be referred have all supporting medical records on your case.
5) Keep copies for yourself of all you medical records.
6) Be prepared to ask your treating physicians questions about your treatment.

SURGICAL PATHOLOGY REPORT

The surgical pathology report is a communication report between physicians. It is a consultation report between the pathologist and the requesting physician. The standard report includes patient demographic information (i.e. Name, location, gender, age, date of birth, physician requesting the evaluation of the tissue, the patient's attending physician and primary physician of record). A pertinent abbreviated clinical history statement is also part of the report as well as identification of the specimen and/or specimens submitted for evaluation, the date and time of the surgery or special procedure, the request for specimen evaluation and the date and time of receipt of the specimen and/or specimens. The pathologist determines the types of specimens received and describes it in the report. The types of breasts specimens or excisions that usually may be received are:

- **Needle Core Biopsies** – cylindrical tissue cores of breast tissue
- **Tylectomy or lumpectomy** - excisional biopsy or surgical removal of breast mass.
- **Quandrantectomy-** removal of one of the four quadrants of the breast.
- **Subcutaneous mastectomy** - removal of the breast tissue without removal of the skin or nipple.
- **Simple (total) mastectomy** - removal of the breast tissue with its skin and nipple.
- **Sentinel node biopsy** - The first lymph node in the group of axillary (underarm) lymph nodes into which lymphatic vessels or channels of the breast drain. If this lymph node is positive for metastatic breast cancer or has tumor in it a complete axillary dissection is usually done.
- **Modified radical mastectomy with axillary node dissection-** removal the breast with some skin and the areola (nipple). Some of the skin is spared for closure of the surgical wound. Lymph nodes with axillary (underarm) fat are also removed.
- **Radical mastectomy** - removal of the entire breast with adjacent adipose (fat) tissue, and chest pectoralis muscles with axillary contents (lymph nodes). This procedure is rarely performed.

- **Supraradical mastectomy** - A radical mastectomy with removal of chest wall and ribs. This procedure is not performed today.

The surgical pathology report includes the weighing, measuring, and gross description and evaluation of the tissue received (i.e. needle biopsies, the removed lump or breast mass, the mastectomy or breast removal or excision). Occasionally radiographs (X-rays) may be taken of lumpectomy specimens received to verify that the area under suspicion has been completely removed. These radiographs may accompany a specimen that have been placed in a Dubin's compression device or a board with a grid. The Dubin's compression device is a round blue plastic container that has a clear circular plastic compressor with a labeled grid. The compressor fits securely in the container and allows the radiologist to compress (apply pressure) to the biopsy. Radiographs are then taken to assure that the suspicious density or calcifications have been removed. The results are relayed to the surgeon and the device with the specimen and radiographs are sent to pathology. The device's grid has holes in it which allow the pathologist to mark the tissue in the area of suspicion with colored ink. After comparing the X and Y axis of the grid with the radiographs, ink marks are placed on the grid holes accordingly. The pathologist can then submit the inked area of suspicion in labeled blocks for processing and evaluation under the microscope.

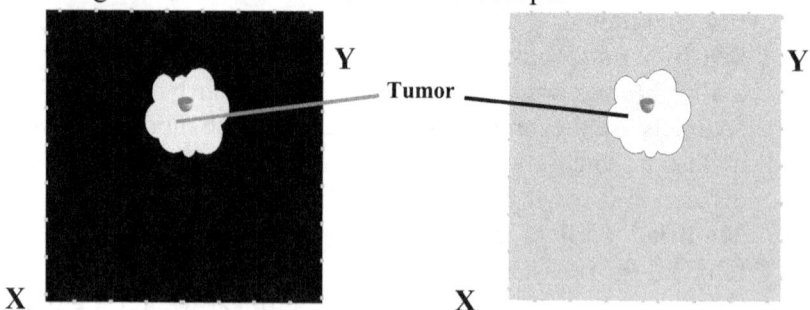

When the pathologist receive any breast specimen, he/she will determine the specimen type and will ink the surgical margins of excision of the specimen with different colored inks and orient the specimen as the marked that the surgeon has placed on it. These are usually different sutures (threads) or metal clip markers which are placed at the margins of excision, the sides and at the top of the removed tissue or breast lump by the surgeon. Any grossly apparent lesions or abnormalities are measured. Any other gross abnormalities and the tissue consistency are described. Any areas which are nodular, calcified, hardened, firm or gritty, are also noted. If the specimen is from a mastectomy the excised breast tumor is evaluated as well as tissue from each quadrant of the breast. Sections of any attached muscle, and all lymph nodes of the axilla (underarm) that are received are usually submitted for evaluation. The dimensions of the lesion or tumor and its distance from the surgical margins of excision are also measured. The specimen is thinly sliced with a sharp knife and multiple sections of the mass or lesion, the tissue adjacent to the tumor or mass and the margins of excision are submitted for processing. After the tissue that has been submitted it is processed overnight The next day slides of the tissue are prepared by the histotechnician and the slides are later reviewed by the pathologist under the microscope.

The surgical pathology contains the following information:
- Specimen type and site
- Specimen size (in three dimensions)
- Tumor size
- Tumor histologic type
- Tumor invasive
- Carcinoma in situ (present or absent) (if percentage is given)
- Tumor grade (all ductal NOS tumors should be graded)
- Tumor necrosis (present or absent)
- The adequacy of surgical margins of excision (free of tumor or not free of tumor)
- Distance of the tumor from the margin of excision
- Presence of multifocal disease
- Presence of tumor extension into blood vessels and lymphatic vessels, or in nerve fibers
- Chest wall involvement
- Skin involvement
– Presence of microcalcifications

   - Metastatic tumor in lymph nodes and the number of lymph nodes
involved
   - The presence of other significant breast disease (atypical duct
hyperplasia or hyperplasia without atypia)
   - Presence of metastases in other organs or tissue sites biopsied
   - Results of ER, PR, HER2, SPF, DNA index, Ki67 and other
studies

The surgeon, primary care physician and consulting physicians can determine by the pathology report the presumptive stage of the cancer by the tumor size and the presence of lymph node metastases and other site involvement. (Refer to previous discussion on TNM Staging and Grading).

The pathologist orders other diagnostic tests on the cancerous breast tissue when indicated, namely, the hormone receptors, **estrogen (ER), and progesterone (PR), and Human Epidermal Growth Factor Receptor 2 (HER2)**, which are prognostically significant tumor markers. Slides are prepared and stained for these receptors. The response of breast tissue to hormones has been known for a long time. ER and PR results are reported as positive or negative. ER and PR are reported as positive is 1% or more of the tumor cell nuclei are staining with the immunohistochemical stain. HER2 is performed directly on the breast tissue. HER2 expression is determined by Immunohistochemistry (IHC) HercepTest which evaluates the level of HER2 protein in the cancer cells. The results are reported as:

> 0 – Negative
> 1+ - Trace/Negative
> 2+ - Weak Positive (staining in >10% of cells)
> 3+ - Strong Positive(staining in >10% of cells)

Any tumor staining which by the HercepTest is scored 1+ referred for testing by Fluorescence in Situ Hybridization (FISH) test. About 70% of breast cancers have positive estrogen receptors (ER) and 60% are positive for progesterone receptor (PR). The results of these tests are usually included on the surgical pathology report.[1] Patient's with ER and/or PR receptor positive tumors have longer disease free survivals. Patients with tumors with overexpression of HER2 or are HER2 + have a poor 5 year survival rates from 15% to 35%. All breast cancers should be tested for ER, PR and HER2.

Flow cytometry is usually ordered. Flow cytometry identifies the cells that are in S-phase or the DNA synthesizing phase of the cell cycle. The cell cycle S-phase fraction (SPF) value and a DNA index are provided. The S-phase fraction (SPF) is an assessment of tumor cell proliferation. The SPF is determined by the intensity of the fluorescence of the DNA of the cells as read by the flow cytometer. Breast cancers' SPF values range from 7% to 13%. Normal cells have an SPF less than 5%. The DNA index compares the DNA content of the tumor cell to that of a normal cell. A DNA index of 1.0 means that the cells are diploid and are similar to normal breast cells in their DNA content. A DNA content that is aneuploid has an abnormal DNA content. A DNA index of 2.0 or more indicates the tumor is hyperdiploid and has abnormal DNA content that is greater then the normal cell. About 70% of breast cancers will be aneuploid and 30% will be diploid. The 5 year disease free survival for women with diploid tumors is 88% and for women with aneuploid tumors is 68%. The 5 year disease free survival for patients with with a diploid tumor and a low SPF is 90% and those with diploid tumors and a high SPF is 70%. Elevated SPF and DNA index is associated with shorter disease free intervals and patient survival times.

Ki67 is a protein or nuclear antigen present in all cells in the non-resting or G_0 phase of the cell cycle. It identifies cells that are proliferating or multiplying in the tumor. The higher the Ki67 growth fraction indicates the more aggressive the tumor. This correlates with the grade of the tumor, the amount of blood vessel invasion and the presence of metastases to lymph nodes. Tumors without lymph nodes metastases typically have Ki67 growth fractions that are less than 10%. Estrogen and progesterone negative tumors usually have a high Ki67 growth fraction.

The following invasive duct carcinomas with a favorable prognosis: tubular, cribiform, medullary, mucinous, papillary, adenoid cystic and juvenile or secretory carcinoma. Tumors with necrosis or degeneration or softening are associated with increased spread to lymph nodes. Tumor involvement of the skin and blood vessels is associated with a poor prognosis.

References:

1. Jones, Stephen E. Update in Hormonal Therapy A 2004 Perspective. Physicians Education Resource. 2004.

Lessons To Be Learned

1) Make sure you obtain a copy of your pathology report either from your physician or directly from the pathology department.
2) Make sure that you discuss the information with your physician so that you can understand the report and make sure that there is enough information to make a decision.
3) What is the type of cancer?
4) What is the grade of the cancer?
5) What is the stage of the cancer?
6) Is there spread of the cancer into the lymph nodes?
7) Is there spread of the cancer into the blood stream?
8) Are other organs involved?
9) What is the prognosis for this cancer?
10) What additional tests were done on the cancer so that treatment decisions can be made?
11) Ask your physician if you are a candidate for breast conservation surgery?
12) Ask whether or not lymph nodes will be removed?
13) If you are told that you need a mastectomy ask if there are other options. Discuss whether or not you are a candidate to have chemotherapy to downstage and reduce the size of the tumor to allow breast conservation surgery.
14) Discuss the possibility of reconstruction surgery ?
15) Ask whether or not you will have to have chemotherapy and or radiation therapy?

CHEMOTHERAPY

Approximately 20% of patients diagnosed with invasive breast cancer in the United States are expected to die of breast cancer. The five year survival rate of patients with local disease or disease confined to the breast is 97%. The five-year survival rate for patients with spread of the tumor to regional lymph nodes is 79% and for those with metastases or spread to a vital organ (liver, lung, brain) is 23%. Although surgery with radiation and chemotherapy has improved survival rates and prognosis for patients. There is still need for improvement.

Chemotherapy works as a treatment by using agents that affect the cell life cycle. The cell life cycle five phases are G_0, $G1$, S, G_2, and M.

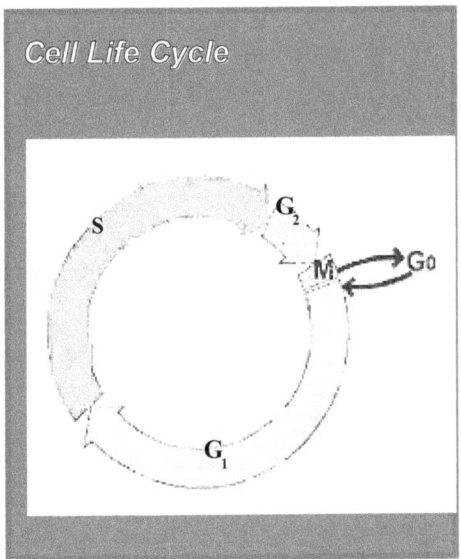

Figure 21-1.

> **Phase G_0- Resting** stage where the cells are not dividing. This may be a few hours or years long.
> **Phase S**- DNA (deoxyribonucleic acid) the hereditary material or genetic content, the instructions or blueprint is made during the S

phase. The chromosomes of the new cell will have the same DNA content or chromosomes as the original cell.

Phase G$_2$ -The mitotic spindle apparatus is constructed. It is a microtubule structure to which the chromosomes are attached and separate to opposite poles of the cell when it divides. The chromosomes line up 2 hrs before the cell splits. This is the period of growth and development and the cell's organelle replication.

Phase M -Mitosis is when the cell splits into two cells. It has the following stages:

Interphase

G$_1$ - The cell begins to grow and develop and makes RNA (ribonucleic acid), the nucleic acid that functions in protein synthesis. The nuclear membrane is intact and the chromosomes of the cell are not visible. The cell prepares for mitosis or cell division.

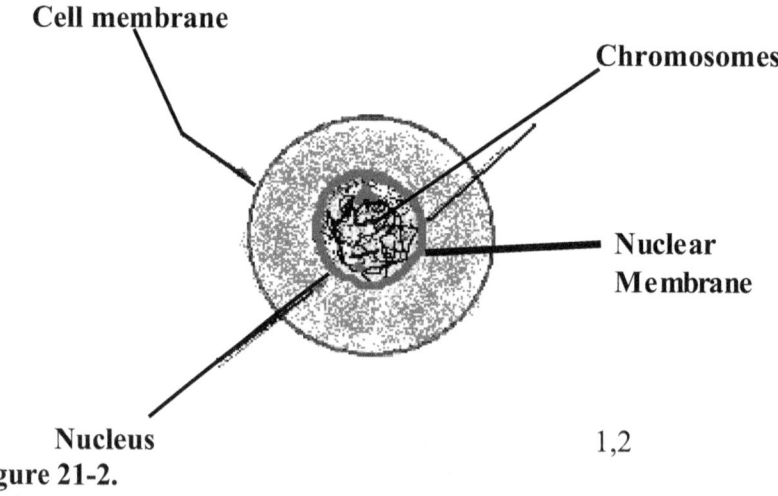

Cell membrane

Chromosomes

Nuclear Membrane

Nucleus   1,2

Figure 21-2.

Prophase - Replicated chromosomes are condensed, supercoiled and compact. The nuclear membrane disperses (disappears). Some fibers cross the cell and begin to form the mitotic spindle.

Figure 21-3.

Centromere 1,2

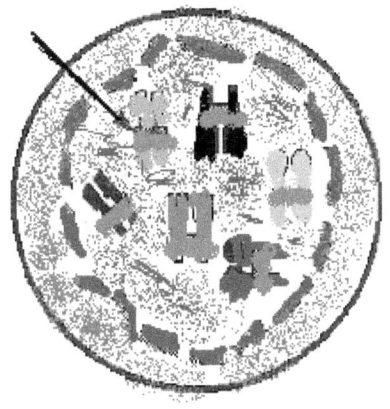

Prometaphase - The nuclear membrane dissolves and spindle fibers form. Proteins attach to centromeres and form kinetochores where

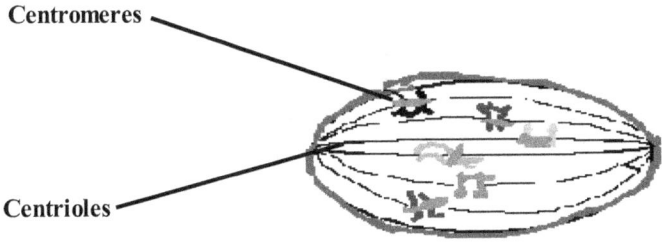

Figure 21-4.
the microtubules are attach. The chromosomes begin to migrate.

Metaphase - The replicated (duplicated) chromosomes align at center in single file on the metaphase equator of the cell or metaphase plate. This ensures that each new cell will have a copy of each chromosome that is identical to the original cell.

Figure 21-5.

Metaphase plane

Metaphase

Centromeres

Centriole

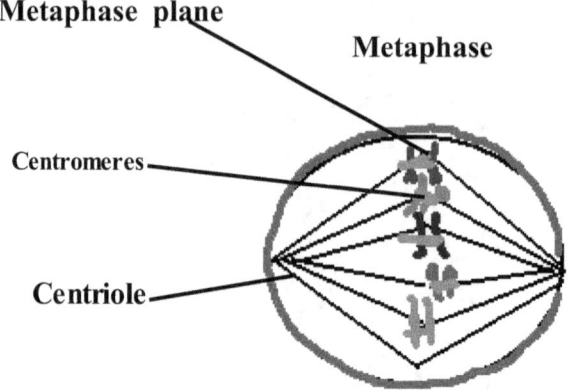

Anaphase - The sister chromosomes separate at the kinetochores and the daughter chromosomes move to opposite sides of the cell.

Figure 21-6.   **Anaphase**

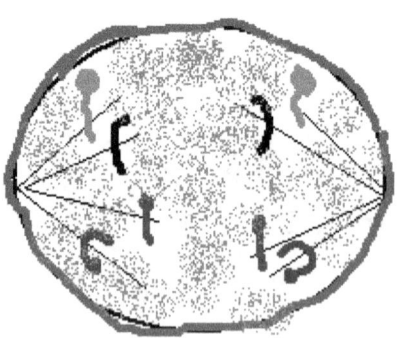

Telophase - New nuclear membranes form around the daughter cell nuclei. The spindle fibers disappear and a cleavage furrow appears while chromosomes reach the poles of the cell.
Figure 21-7.

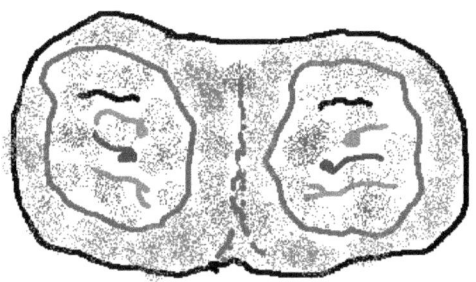

Telophase

Cytokinesis: The cell divides into two daughter cells as the chromosomes disappear. Chromatin reforms and the cells enter the G1 or resting phase.
Figure 21-8.

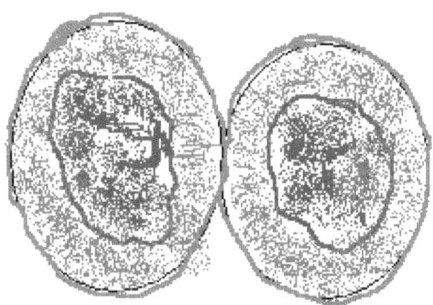

Cytokinesis

The physician's goal is to cure the patient by killing the cancer cells. Knowledge of the cell cycle is important in order to disrupt the growth of cancer cells. Chemotherapy drugs work on reproducing cancer cells in their S or M phase by interrupting the cell cycle and destroying the cell. The chemotherapy drugs used cannot distinguish between cancer cells and normal cells; therefore all cells in the body, normal cells and cancer cells alike, that is in either the S or M phase are also affected. This is the unwanted side effect of chemotherapy treatment.

Chemotherapy drugs may be given as neoadjuvants, which are drugs that are used with or without radiation to shrink the tumor before surgery so that the tumor can be removed. Neoadjuvants are effective in shrinking estrogen receptor (ER) negative breast cancers. Neoadjuvants are more effective in breast cancers with low estrogen receptor (ER) levels and are less effective on breast cancers that have high estrogen receptor (ER) levels. Chemotherapy drugs are also given as adjuvant agents, (i.e. hormonal therapy drugs or other drugs) used in chemotherapy, in order to prevent the growth of remaining cancer cells prior to radiation and after surgery.

The physician or oncologist will determine how to best treat a patient. Treatment will be based upon the stage of disease and the tumor biologic subtype as ER+/HER2+ or ER-/HER2-, and whether or not the patient is premenopausal, peri-menopausal or postmenopausal. The patient's age and life expectancy is also taken into consideration as well as any disease states which might limit whether or not the patient can tolerate treatment. If there is no significant disease factors that would limit the patient's ability to undergo chemotherapy treatment safely, the patient should receive treatment. Ageism still is a factor in treating older women and they sometimes go undertreated. This results in poor disease free intervals and overall survival in these patients. Older women should discuss their therapy, life expectancy and other health conditions with their physician to be sure that they receive the right treatment. In stage I and II, lymph node negative breast cancer patients with tumors that are ER+ HER2-, breast cancer multigene assays like Oncotype DX, Mammaprint or PAM50 may be used to predict the chemotherapy benefit by determining whether or not a patient is at low risk for recurrence or at high risk for recurrence. Patients who are low risk can be treated with hormonal therapy alone and high risk patients should receive both hormone therapy and chemotherapy. Patients with stage III or locally advanced disease 66% to 90% will be lymph node positive. Neoadjuvant chemotherapy (chemotherapy prior to surgery) can be given to downstage the disease so that the tumor can be made operable so that the patient can either have breast conserving therapy or mastectomy followed by radiation therapy. Treatment for stage III disease is a multimodality approach involving pre-operative chemotherapy, followed by surgery and radiation therapy.

When breast cancer is at an advanced stage, Stage IV, the physician will try to control the advancement of the disease to extend the patient's life. Stage IV disease is advanced metastatic disease which may include metastases to bone, brain, spinal cord, lung, liver and other sites. Radiation is the mainstay of treatment and is palliative. Surgery for removal of brain metastases, spinal cord compression lesions, the stabilization of fractures and procedures to remove the accumulation of fluid in the space around the lungs and heart or the removal of metastatic tumor deposits in the gastrointestinal tract is in no means curative but may be beneficial to the patient's quality of life. When tumor control is impossible because of the extent of the disease, then the physician will try to control the pain and symptoms of the advanced disease, using palliative treatment to improve the quality of life for the time that is left.

It is imperative that as a patient you understand your treatment plans and ask questions. You and your spouse or caretaker or friend, should make sure that the important questions are asked. Ask the physician what you can expect with chemotherapy. Ask whether or not you will be cured of the disease. Know what medications you will be given and how they will be given. Ask for the regimen on how often the drugs will be given. Ask whether or not it may affect your work or if you can continue to work. Ask what type of limitations will be placed on your daily activities and whether or not you need someone to take you to your office visits or to assist you at home. Ask what the side effects of each drug are and what will be done to reduce these side effects. Ask whether or not there are any long-term side effects that you may have for taking the drugs. Ask what side effects are considered serious enough to discontinue the treatment. Ask the doctor whom you may contact if you need to ask a question or have an emergent condition and need to be seen.

Chemotherapy drugs may be given intravenously (infused in the vein) or given orally. The most commonly drugs used for Her2-negative and Her2-positive tumors and for women with recurrent and or metastatic disease are: Adriamycin (Doxorubicin), Cytoxan (Cyclophosphamide), Ellence(Epirubicin), Navelbine(Vinorelbine), Taxol (Paclitaxel), Taxotere (Docetaxel), Xeloda (Capecitabine), and Gemzar (Gemcitabine). These drugs may be given as single agents but are usually used in various combinations. The drugs are usually given in cycles and followed by a rest period before the next cycle. The most common regimens follow.

Her2-negative tumor chemotherapy drugs:

- Adriamycin or (Epirubicin) followed by cyclophosamide/methotrexate/fluorouracil**(CMF)**
    {A or (E)-->CMF}
- Doxorubicin/cyclophosphamide**(AC)**   followed by paclitaxel four times every two weeks **{AC x 4-->Tx4}** or
- Doxorubicin followed by paclitaxel followed by cyclophosphamide every two weeks **{A-->T-->C}**.

Her2-positive tumor chemotherapy drugs:

- **(AC)** is followed by Paclitaxel with Trastuzumab as an adjuvant **{AC-->T+Trastuzumab}**or
- Paclitaxel plus trastuzumab followed by Cyclophosamide/Epirubicin/Fluorouracil **(CEF)** plus Trastuzumab **{T+ Trastuzumab-->CEF +Trastuzumab}** may be given as a neoadjuvant before surgery.

Preferred combination therapies with Trastuzumab:

- Trastuzumab with Paclitaxel with or without carboplatin
- Trastuzumab with Docetaxel with or without carboplatin or
- Trastuzumab with Vinorelbine.

Current treatment for regional (local) and extensive disease (disease involving or spreading to other organs, lymph nodes and bone) requires classical chemotherapy agents. Chemotherapy is not new. Physicians have been using such agents for over 30 years to help benefit patients and to help improve the disease free interval (time) and overall survival of patients. The drugs have been studied through the use of clinical trials to help identify the best regimens. Clinical trials are health-related research studies using humans to investigate a treatment.

Researchers have studied the use of anthracycline and non-anthracycline drug regimens based on the HER2 receptor status of patients. One such study of 18,000 women under age 50 with lymph node negative disease showed a 7% benefit with a 10-year survival rate. Another study involving women over age 50 showed an improved survival rate of 2%. The study used an anthracycline regimen versus cyclophosamide/methotextrate/5-fluorouracil (CMF) regimen in which there was an additional 3% benefit with a 5 yr survival rate. Current therapies for breast cancer treatment are based on the evidence received from such clinical trials or studies. At present several different regimens of chemotherapy exist, however there are no predictive markers for an individual patient's response to these regimens. What we do know for certain however is that patients who are lymph node negative or without tumor in their lymph nodes and whose tumors are ER negative with HER2 overexpression (ER-/HER2+) are at high risk for recurrence of breast cancer and should receive an anthracycline based chemotherapy regimen with an alkylating agent. [3,4]

More recent trials that are attempting to determine whether or not the change in sequencing and scheduling and dosing of the drugs may alter patient survival outcome.[5] One such study involved a sequential form of chemotherapy for early stage breast cancer where chemotherapy drugs were given in cycles following each other had better outcomes than two shorter regimens given concurrently or at the same time in four cycles.[6] Doxorubicin/Cyclophosamide given in four cycles followed by Taxotere for four cycles given sequentially was the better regimen. This is why most breast cancer patients with risk for recurrence receive four courses of Adriamycin or Epirubicin 90mg/m2 plus Cytoxan or Cyclophosphamide 600mg/m2 followed by 4 courses of Taxol or Paclitaxel 175 mg/m2.

Another study done by Sparano el al in their recent study found that giving Paclitaxel weekly during the chemotherapy treatment had significant better survival rate and improved disease free interval compared to the administration of Paclitaxel every three weeks.[7]

It has been common practice in the past to give patients with advanced metastatic disease the same drugs as patients with less advanced disease, but now new therapeutic regimens and strategies using the drugs Fluoropyrimidine, Capecitabine and the Vinca alkaloid Vinorelbine are being studied and evaluated when combined with the taxanes and/or the anthracylines.[8] Patients with Her2/neu overexpression (Her2+) that have failed chemotherapy may now receive this treatment and have an objective response rate of 15%. Studies using Trastuzumab (anti-Her2) with various combinations of chemotherapeutic drugs continue to be performed. When Trastuzumab is used first line for metastatic breast cancer, the response rate varies from 26% when used as a single agent to 75% when used with the drugs docetaxel and vinorelbine. There is now a second line therapy for recurrent metastatic breast cancer that consists of treatment with Gemcitabine and Trastuzumab that shows a 38% response rate.

Table 21-1. Trastuzumab-Chemotherapy Combinations

Chemotherapy	*N*	*Response Rate*
First-lineMetastaticBreastCancer		
Single-agent T	114	26%
Doxorubicin + T	30	55%
Vinorelbine + T	69	61%
Gemcitabine + P + T	42	67%
Docetaxel + vinorelbine + T	29	75%
Second-line or Later Metastatic Breast Cancer		
Gemcitabine + T	61	38%

It is expected that as more clinical trials are completed there will be continued improvement in chemotherapy and treatment management. If you decide to participate in a clinical trial know that by contributing to such research studies you are helping others in the future. There are strict medical ethical and legal codes that govern clinical trials to protect you as a participant. If you doctor wants to you to be a participant, be sure to ask you doctor questions about the trial and ask him what your protections are as a participant.

COMMON CHEMOTHERAPEUTIC AGENTS USED IN BREAST CANCER TREATMENT

Doxorubicin (Adriamycin) is an antineoplastic drug that interferes with the growth of cancer cells and normal body cells. It is administered intravenously and may cause unusual allergic reactions and birth defects in the fetus if administered to a mother during pregnancy. Breast-feeding is not recommended. This drug may cause heart, cardiac toxicities in young children and the elderly who are more sensitive to the drug. The **most common adverse effects** of Doxorubicin are:
- hair loss
- headache
- hypotension (low blood pressure)
- nausea and vomiting
- leukopenia (low white blood cell count)
- thrombocytopenia (low platelet count)
- anemia
- chills
- diarrhea
- facial edema (face swelling)
- weakness

Other less frequent effects are allergic reactions, back pain, cardiotoxicity (heart toxicity) i.e. (heart conduction defects, fast heart beat and irregular heart beat), constipation, dizziness, drug fever, difficulty swallowing, redness of the palms and soles and other parts of the skin, itching of the skin and skin rashes, scaling of the feet and hands, and skin swelling.

It is up to you to make sure that your healthcare provider is made aware of any other medications that you may be taking that can interfere with or cause adverse reactions while taking Doxorubicin (Adriamycin). This includes over the counter medications, vitamins, nutriments and alternative drugs. Make sure that your physician knows everything you are taking particularly the following medically prescribed drugs or therapies: Amphotericin, antithyroid medications, Azathioprine or Imuran, Chloramphenicol, Colchicine, Flucytosine, Ganciclovir, Interferon, Plicamycin, Zidovudine or AZT, Retrovir, previous radiation, Probenecid and Sulfinpyrazone. Make sure that you let your doctor know if you have gout, since Doxorubicin increases uric acid levels and may cause kidney stones. Let your physician know if you have any type of heart problems because the drug may cause cardiac or heart toxicities. The drug may also affect the liver since it is metabolized and removed from the body very slowly. If you have a history of chronic anemia or low white blood cell count, platelet count or an infection of any kind, be sure that your doctor is aware of these conditions because it may possibly be significant in your treatment plans.

The drug Doxorubicin together with Cyclophosamide is the standard chemotherapy regimen for breast cancer.[9] If you receive these drugs and your tumor only has a partial response to the treatment it may be because your tumor is resistant or insensitive to the drug. There are specific genes that regulate the metabolism of cells, protein synthesis and estrogen related pathways that may make the tumor cells resistant to the drug. [1] There are reference laboratories that do testing on tumor cells to determine their sensitivity to combinations of chemotherapy drugs and your physician should be aware of this.

Epirubicin is one of the most active antineoplastic agents used for breast cancer. It also interferes with the growth of normal cells as well as cancer cells and is metabolized by the liver. In the planning of treatment with your doctor be sure to ask about the drugs side effects. The major **side effects of Epirubicin** are:
- alopecia (hair loss)
- amenorrhea (loss of menstrual period)

- anemia(low red cell count)
- bone marrow depression
- esophagitis (inflammation of the esophagus)
- infections
- leukopenia (low white blood cell count)
- nausea and vomiting
- stomatitis (inflammation of the oral cavity or mouth)
- discolored urine
- abscess (accumulates pus)
- diarrhea
- ulcers of the stomach and intestines
-hyperuricemia (increased uric acid in the blood)
-phlebitis (inflammation of the veins)
- postirradiation erythema (redness of the skin after radiation)
- low platelet count
- thrombophlebitis (inflammation and blood clots in the veins)
- necrosis or degeneration of tissue or flesh
- gout and kidney disorder from uric acid accumulation in the blood and tissues
- blood vessel spasms associated with menopause (hot flashes)

Rarely acute myeloid leukemia occurs if a high dose regimen is used. [10] Allergic reactions, anorexia (lack of appetite), chills and fever, itching of skin, skin rash and skin thickening, chronic heart failure and heart toxicity may occur.[11] Be sure to let your physician know if you have any history of heart disease of any type, if you are pregnant or nursing or have a history of bone marrow or blood disorders, kidney disease or infection. Such conditions are contraindications for the use of this drug.

If this drug is used in your treatment plan, contact your physician if you experience any bleeding, ulcers or sores in the mouth or throat, cough or hoarseness, irregular heart beat, fever or chills, back or side pain, painful or difficult urination, bruising or bleeding in the skin, black tarry stools, red spots on the skin, redness of the eye or discharge of the eye, redness of the skin at the radiation site, skin rash or itching, belly swelling, or swelling of the feet and lower legs, enlarged lymph glands, shortness of breath, a high fever or swelling of the lining of the mouth, nose or throat.

Cyclophosamide (Cytoxan) is an antineoplastic used in breast cancer and is a first line therapy drug or first drug of choice used for treatment of breast cancer. It is also used to treat other cancers, i.e. Tumors of the blood and lymphatic system (lymphomas, multiple myeloma, leukemias, mycosis fungoides), neuroblastoma, ovarian cancers, retinoblastoma (eye cancer in children) and autoimmune disorders. Make sure your physician knows if you are a nursing mother, pregnant, dehydrated (have lost a lot of fluid) or have a blood and bone marrow disorder. Doxorubicin induced cardiomyopathy (heart disease), hemorrhagic induced cystitis (inflammation of the bladder), viral, bacterial, fungal, parasitic or protozoal infections, kidney disorders and stones, gout and liver disease or allergies to this drug. Let your physician know if you have had any recent vaccinations to measles or flu shots, or if you have had chemotherapy before. The use of the drug is contraindicated in these conditions.

The **adverse effects** of this drug are:
- abdominal pain and cramps
- alopecia (hair loss) and brittle and thin hair
- infections
- irregular menstrual periods
- leukopenia (low white count)
- darkened skin and nails
- nausea and vomiting
- skin thickening and blistering
- fatigue
- pericarditis (inflammation around the heart and heart sac)
- anemia
- thrombocytopenia (low platelet count)
- uric acid kidney disease and gout
- nephrotoxicity (kidney toxicity)
- hepatitis(liver inflammation)
- bronchospasms or lung spasms
- pulmonary (lung) disease
- shortness of breath
- hyperhidrosis (excess sweating)
- hyperglycemia (high blood sugar)
- allergic reactions with swelling of face

- urticaria (hives)
- skin rashes and itching
- stomatitis (inflammation of the mouth or oral cavity)

It is imperative that you drink plenty of fluids during the first 24 hours after treatment. If you experience any of the following symptoms while on Cyclophosamide, like pain on urination or red urine, black tarry stools, unusual bleeding or bruising, cough and congestion, fever and chills, shortness of breath, sore mouth and blisters, swelling of the feet or ankles, excessive nausea and vomiting or a rash contact you physician immediately.

Docetaxel is an antineoplastic drug used in combination with other drugs to treat breast cancer. It is also used in the treatment of non-small cell cancer of lung, prostate cancer, bladder cancer, esophageal cancer, head and neck cancer, ovarian cancer and stomach cancer.[12]. It acts by interfering with cell growth. It is administered intravenously.

Docetaxel should not be used if you have allergies or are sensitive to the drug, are pregnant or breast-feeding, or in the elderly. Make sure your physician knows all other drugs and over the counter medications that you may be taking because some of these drugs may be contraindicated while using Docetaxel. Docetaxel may also increase the effects of radiation therapy on the red and white cells of the blood and platelets. While using some antibiotics i.e. erythromycin or antifungal medications, the blood levels of Docetaxel may increase and cause toxic effects. No immunizations should be given while you are on this drug without you doctor's consent. Make sure that your physician knows if you have a history of alcohol abuse, liver disease, bacterial, fungal, or viral infection. Your doctor should be notified immediately if any of the following symptoms occur: fever or chills, cough, voice hoarseness, back or side pain, pain on urination, bleeding or brusing, black stools, bloody urine, and red spots on your skin. Do not touch your eyes before washing your hands. Do not pick your nose, cut yourself or play contact sports. You are at an increased risk for bleeding and infections while on this drug. The most common **adverse effects** of the drug are:
- swelling of the abdomen face, fingers, hands, feet and lower legs

- weight gain
- tiredness and weakness

Other less common side effects are severe red scaling areas of the skin, decreased in blood pressure, fainting and dizziness, or increase in blood pressure with headaches and dizziness.

If your physician puts you Docetaxel be sure to keep scheduled appointments. Your physician will routinely check you at each office visit for anemia and low white blood cell count, blood platelet count, changes in blood pressure. You should also notify your physician if any additional side effects occur, like burning sensations, numbness and tingling or pain in arms, legs, feet, congestion, diarrhea sore throat, nausea, red skin rash and redness of the palms and soles with scaling, mouth ulcers and weakness in legs, arms, hands or feet, bloody nose, body aches and pains, nail color changes, swollen eyes and eyelids, hives, stomach pain, wrinkled skin, swollen neck glands, difficulty swallowing, pain all over the body, muscles and joints with a runny nose.

Paclitaxel (Taxol) is an antineoplastic agent or drug used in locally advanced and metastatic breast cancer treatment. It is also used in the treatment of Kaposi's sarcoma, non-small carcinoma of lung, ovarian carcinoma, bladder cancer, carcinomas of the head and neck, Non-Hodgkin's lymphoma, small cell lung carcinoma and carcinoma in situ of the esophagus. Paclitaxel is administered intravenously. It interferes with the growth of cancer cells by affecting the mitotic spindle apparatus of the cell and cause the cells to vibrate.

If you are breast feeding, pregnant or want to become pregnant, have a low white cell or platelet count or have bone marrow disorders, clotting disorders, liver disease, neurological disorders (Parkinson's disease or peripheral nerve damage), severe bacterial, fungal or protozoal infection, abnormal ECG, angina or heart failure tell your physician because the use of this drug may be contraindicated in these conditions. Tell your doctor if you are taking the following medications: Amphotericin B, antithyroid agents, Azathioprine (Imuran), Chloramphenicol, Colchicine, Flucytosine, Ganciclovir, Interferon, Plicamycin, or AZT. If you have had recent exposure to chickenpox, or have herpes virus, heart problems or other

infections, please let your physician know.
The **adverse effects** of Paclitaxel are:

- allergic reactions and dermatitis
- alopecia
- anemia
- leukopenia
- arthralgia (joint pain)
- diarrhea
- nausea and vomiting
- shortness of breath
- weakness
- peripheral nerve damage
- skin rashes and
- erythema (reddening of skin)
- liver dysfunction
- hypotension (low blood pressure)
- abscess
- phlebitis
- stomatitis

The use of this drug mandates that you check in with your doctor when scheduled so that unwanted side effects can be discovered. Do not have any immunizations without your doctors approval because you might develop a superinfection. Avoid people with infections. If you notice unusual bleeding, bruising, black tarry stools, blood in your stools or urine, red spots on your skin, cough or hoarseness, chills, fever, lower back or side pain, shortness of breath, redness at drug injection sites, and sores on your mouth or lips contact your doctor. Do not engage in contact sports. Be careful in cleaning your teeth and gums. Wash your hands frequently. Do not touch your eyes or the insides of your nose unless you have washed your hands. Do not cut yourself with sharp objects.

Trastuzumab (Herceptin) is a recombivant monoclonal antibody against HER2 used in the treatment of high-risk node negative breast cancers and metastatic breast cancers that have HER2 overexpression. Multiple clinical trials have shown a clear therapeutic benefit of using Trastuzumab with the chemotherapy regimen.[13]   Trastuzumab is not associated with the adverse effects that occur with chemotherapy, however, hypersensitivity to Trastuzumab has been known to occur as well as congestive heart failure.[17] It is not known whether or not Trastuzumab increases heart toxicity when administered with other chemotherapy drugs which cause heart toxicity.

If you are pregnant or breast feeding, have had heart dysfunction after having a heart attack or have congestion of the lung and severe shortness of breath or a lung condition, this drug should not be used. The most common **adverse reactions** are:

- dizziness
- fever and/or chills
- headache
- nausea and/or vomiting
- shortness of breath
- skin rash
- weakness

Rare adverse reactions that may occur are adult respiratory distress syndrome (ARDS), allergic reactions, anaphylaxis (low blood pressure with circulatory collapse), angioedema (body swelling), hypoxia (lack of oxygen to the body), pleural effusions (fluid in the chest), pulmonary edema (fluid in the lungs), respiratory depression, itching of skin and urticaria (hives). Rarely there may be tightness in the chest, troubled breathing and wheezing. You should immediately notify your physician if you experience irregular heartbeat, increased cough, swelling of the feet and legs, blue lips and fingers, blurred vision, chest pain, cough or hoarseness, fever and chills, light headedness when standing, a hive like reaction of the face, eyelids, lips, tongue, throat, hands and feet, sex organs, lower side or back pain, chills and fever, painful urination, pale skin, redness of the skin and tiredness or weakness.

Bevacizumab(Avastin) is also a recombivant **humanized monoclonal antibody and anti-tumor agent.** It is a targeted agent and has been used in combination with standard chemotherapy as part of the first line therapy for patients with metastatic breast cancer and is used in combination with Paclitaxel for the initial treatment of metastatic HER2-

negative breast cancer. Recent studies have shown that patients receiving Avastin do not have significant progression free survival, overall survival and higher response rate to therapy as in previous studies. Recently it was recommended that Avastin no longer be used in the treatment of breast cancer. The drug has been associated with the following **adverse effects**:
- hypertension
- protein in the urine
- decreased nerve sensation
- heart dysfunction
- perforations of the stomach and intestines[14]

Vinorelbine is an antineoplastic agent or drug used in the treatment of metastatic breast cancer. It is a vinca alkaloid. Its use is not indicated in patients who have bone marrow depression or who may be pregnant. The most frequent **adverse effects** of Vinorelbine are:
- alopecia (hair loss)
- anemia
- constipation
- fatigue
- weakness
- leukopenia (low white cell count)
- nausea and vomiting
- nerve damage (numbness)
- phlebitis (inflammation of veins)
- anorexia (loss of appetite)
- arthralgia (joint pain)
- chest pain
- diarrhea
- jaw pain
- myalgia (muscle pain)
- stomatitis (inflammation of the mouth or oral cavity)
- paralytic ileus (paralyzed small bowel or loss of bowel motility)
- thrombocytopenia (low platelets)

Let your physician know if you have a history of blood or bone marrow disorder, a current infection (viral or bacterial), and are pregnant or nursing or have lung disease. [10]

Gemcitabine (Gemzar) is an antimetabolic drug used in breast cancer and other kinds of malignancy that interferes with the growth of the cancer cells and normal cells. It is administered intravenously. Tell your physician if you have any allergies to the drug, or are pregnant or nursing. Let your healthcare provider know if you have a history of or have been recently exposed to chicken pox or have shingles. Let your physician know if you have a kidney disease or liver disease. Let your physician know if you are taking the following medications Azathioprine (Imuran), Chlorambucil (Leukeran), steroids, Cyclosporine, Mercaptopurine, Muromonab-CD3 or Tacrolimus (Progaf), which may put you at increased risk to developing infection.

Gemcitabine lowers the white blood cell count and the platelet count. While you are on the drug you are at an increased risk for infection. You should avoid people with infections. If you develop tarry black stools, cough or hoarseness, shortness of breath, noisy breathing, lower back or side pain, blood in the urine or stools, red spots on your skin, yellow eyes and decrease urination, please notify your healthcare provider. Wash your hands often. Do not touch your eyes or the inside of your nose or cut yourself while shaving or caring for your nails. Do not play rough sports, which can cause bruising, or injury. The most common **adverse reactions** are:

- constipation
- diarrhea
- general illness
- anorexia (appetite loss)
- myalgia (muscle pain)
- nausea and vomiting
- rhinorrhea (runny noise)
- sweating
- trouble sleeping

Irritation, excessive drowsiness, numbness and tingling of the hands and feet, sores and ulcers and white spots on the lips and in the mouth may occur. Rare adverse reactions like serious allergic reactions with reddened face, rash, hives or itching, puffiness of face and eyelids may occur. If this happens you should see your doctor immediately.

Gemcitabine is usually used in hormone insensitive breast cancer or breast cancer that is HER2 positive and ER negative. It is used less often than Capecitabine and Vinorelbine but its usage will probably increase in the future. Recent Phase II trials have shown response rates of 14% to 37% and survival up to a year and a half year in patients treated with Gemcitabine.[11] When Docetaxel and Gemcitabine were given as a regimen 79% of patients responded to therapy. The most common adverse effect of patients treated was neutropenia (low white blood cell count). [15]

Tamoxifen(Novaldex) is a selective estrogen receptor modulator (SERM). It has estrogen agonist-antagonist properties. It is an anti-estrogens used in the treatment of breast cancer. It blocks the effects of estrogen in the body by binding to the estrogen receptor and exposing a binding site that is activated by a coactivating protein not used by the estrogen-activated receptor. The drug is used in post cancer treatment and also in premenopausal women who have a high risk of developing breast cancer in order to reduce their risk of developing cancer. If you are considering the use of this drug to reduce your risks for developing breast cancer, be sure to discuss your risks with your physician.

Factors that may increase your risk for breast cancer are:
- A family history of breast cancer in mother, sister or daughter
- Previous breast biopsy with high-risk changes
- Having never been pregnant or having had a late age first pregnancy.
- Having your first period at an early age.

If you think that you may be a candidate for Tamoxifen for the prevention of breast cancer, discuss it with your physician. You should not be on this drug if you have known allergies to Tamoxifen, are breast-feeding or are older and taking many medications. Let your physician know if you are taking any over the counter medications which may interact with Tamoxifen. If your physician places you on Tamoxifen to reduce your risk for breast cancer, take it as directed by your doctor. The dosage that you are prescribed is the exact amount of the medicine that you should take each day and it should not be stopped, even if you feel

nauseous. Make sure your physician knows any side effects that your may be experiencing, so that he can determine ways to lessen these side effects. Make sure that you notify your physician of vaginal discharge, problems with your vision,
coughing up blood, swollen legs or pain, irregular menstrual periods, vaginal bleeding, breast lumps, pelvic or chest pain. and shortness of breath, yellow eyes or skin, weakness, sleepiness, blisters and peeling or loosening of skin and mouth mucous membranes, a hive-like rash, abdominal pain, red skin lesions.

If you are currently on blood thinners and medicines that damage cells your physician should be made aware of the fact. Tamoxifen may affect the eyes and increase your blood cholesterol levels. It has also been known to produce blood clots, pulmonary embolism (blood clots to the lung), strokes and uterine cancer.

The major **adverse effects are:**
- loosening of the skin and mucous membranes
- leg swelling
- cough
- dizziness
- fast heartbeat
- lightheadedness.

The **minor adverse effects** of Tamoxifen are:
- bone pain
- nausea and vomiting
- black tarry stools
- bloody urine
- dry skin
- itching
- confusion
- decrease amount of urine
- hot flashes and warmness of the face, neck and arms
- profuse sweating
- weight gain

Men who are on Tamoxifen may have decrease interest in sex, poor penile erection and decrease sex drive. The drug may also cause hair thinning and hair loss.

Patients with deep vein thrombosis (blood clots), pregnancy and breast feeding, significant lung disease, visual changes and cataracts, low blood white cell count, low blood platelets and high serum cholesterol and lipids should not take this drug.

Letrazole (Femara) is an aromatase inhibitor drug that is taken daily orally. Femara is used for the treatment of steroid hormone receptor positive and early metastatic breast cancer in postmenopausal women. The following are contraindications for the use of this drug: pregnancy, lactation or breast-feeding, osteoporosis, osteopenia, liver disease, high blood cholesterol and the use of Anastrozole. The **adverse effects** of this drug are:

- abdominal pain and cramps
- alopecia (hair loss)
- anxiety
- depression
- arthralgia (joint pain) and arthritis
- constipation
- diarrhea
- drowsiness
- dyspnea (shortness of breath)
- fatigue and weakness
- insomnia
- hyperhidrosis (increased sweating)
- headaches
- hypertension
- limb pain
- myalgia (muscle pain)
- pruritus (itching) of skin
- hot flashes
- nausea and vomiting
- weight gain
- skin rashes
- abnormal liver function
- ECG changes
- blurred vision

- influenza
-excessive menstruation
-osteopenia and osteoporosis (bone loss)
-blood clotting disorders
-urinary tract infections

Letrazole has been found to be slightly more effective than Tamoxifen in a Breast International Group 1-98 Collaborative Group study of roughly 8,000 postmenopausal women where the five year disease free survival was 84% for Letrozole and 81.4% for Tamoxifen. The effect was also better in patients who received chemotherapy. Patients also experienced fewer tendencies to thromboembolism or developing blood clots as well as fewer tendencies to develop endometrial hyperplasia and endometrial carcinoma of the uterus.[16]   Cardiac or heart adverse effects were similar for both Letrazole and Tamoxifen. However, Letrazole was associated with a higher rate of fractures than Tamoxifen. A longer follow-up is needed to see whether or not the risk of cancer recurrence or relapse is further reduced by Letrazole after therapy.[17,18]

Raloxifene (Evista) in a large trial study of 19,747 women has been found to be equivalent to Tamoxifen in its effectiveness and its ability to prevent invasive breast cancer in women with invasive estrogen receptor positive tumors that are at a high risk for the disease. Raloxifene showed a reduction of hip fractures, endometrial hyperplasia of the uterus, osteoporosis (bone loss), thromboembolism (blood clots) and toxic effects.

When deciding to use this medication be sure that your physician knows whether you are pregnant or breast feeding and if you have had any allergic reactions to Raloxifene. The following medications should not be taken with Raloxifene: Cholestyramine (Questran), estrogens of any kind, including the patch, Coumadin (Warfarin). Make your doctor aware of your past medical history and tell your physician if you have a tendency to form blood clots, have had deep vein thrombosis, cancer or other tumors, liver disease and congestive heart failure.

The most common adverse effects of this drug are:
- bloody or cloudy urine
- chest pain
- difficult or painful burning on urination
- infection
- body aches and pains
- runny nose
- congestion in throat
- cough
- dryness or soreness of throat
- loss of voice
- leg cramping
- skin rash
- swelling of hands or feet
- vaginal itching

You should stop taking Evista and consult your physician immediately if you start coughing up blood, have a severe headache, loss of speech, coordination, vision, chest pain, arm or leg pain and shortness of breath.

Epoetin Alfa (Procrit) is a drug used for the treatment of anemia that is the result of chemotherapy and radiation therapy in patients with breast cancer and other non-myeloid cancers. It is erythropoietin, a glycoprotein (starch protein) that stimulates the production of red blood cells and decreases the need for blood transfusions. It may be given as subcutaneous injections (in the fat under the skin) or intravenously (in the vein). Your physician will closely monitor you hemoglobin during treatment. Dosages will be increased or decrease based upon those laboratory results.

The main side effects are that of fever, diarrhea, nausea and vomiting, swelling, weakness and fatigue, shortness of breath, upper respiratory infection, dizziness, trunk and bone pain, and headaches.[19]

Neupogen (Filgrastin) is a human granulocyte (white blood cell) granulocyte colony stimulating factor (G-CSF) used for the treatment of leukopenia or low white blood cell count which is a major side effect of chemotherapy in cancer patients with breast cancer other cancers. It is used for the prevention of infections when white blood cell counts are low. It decreases the need for hospitalization and antibiotics. It is given as subcutaneous injections or intravenously. It is usually administered after the administration of chemotherapy and given daily for up to 2 weeks. Your physician will monitor your white blood cell count.

Neupogen use is contraindicated in patients allergic to E.Coli proteins, or in patients with Sickle cell disease, and low white blood cell count due to some white blood cell neoplastic disorders. The main side **effects** are minor nausea and vomiting, bone pain, hair loss, diarrhea, fever, inflammation of mucosa in mouth, tiredness, loss of appetite, shortness of breath, headaches, cough, skin rash, chest pain and constipation. [20]

Table 21-2. 183

Chemotherapeutic Drugs Used in Breast Cancer Treatment

TREATMENT OF SIDE EFFECTS OF CHEMOTHERAPY

SYMPTOMS	TREATMENT
Alopecia	Cessation of chemotherapy
Allergic reactions	Corticosteroids, Benadryl
Anemia	Procrit
Leukopenia	Neupogen
Arthralgia (joint pain)	Tylenol or Advil, NSAIDs
Diarrhea	Treatment of infection with antibiotics and fluid replacement
Nausea and vomiting	Antiemetics, Benadryl, Lorazepam
Shortness of breath	Exam for lung and heart disease, pulmonary disease,pneumonia, embolism, cardiotoxicity, MI
Weakness	Access diet and rest
Peripheral nerve damage	Glutamine with oxidizers
Skin rashes	Antibiotics, Antifungal or steroid cremes, supportive care
Erythema of skin	Rule out infection, antibiotics, supportive care, steroids
Liver dysfunction	Evaluation of liver disease
Hypotension	Treatment of causes cardiovascular, infection and fluid loss
Abscess	Incision and drainage and antibiotics
Phlebitis	Antibiotics, antitoxin
Stomatitis (mouth infection)	Mouth rinses

Abdominal cramps	Rule out food poisoning or infection, antibiotics
Irregular menstrual periods	Cessation of chemotherapy, check platelet count
Nail discoloration and thickening	Cessation of chemotherapy
Fatigue	Rest and/or treatment of anemia
Esophagitis	Anti-acids and or antifungals
Discolored urine	Rule out blood in urine
Painful urination	Antibiotics for infection
Hyperuricemia (gout)	Colchicine
Stomach ulcers	Anti-acids
Pericarditis	Antibiotics, corticosteroids
Thrombocytopenia	Platelets

CHEMOTHERAPY ADVERSE DRUG REACTIONS Table 21-3.

DRUG	REACTIONS
Doxorubicin	Hairloss, headache, hypotension, nausea, vomiting, leukopenia, nausea, vomiting, low platelets, anemia, chills, diarrhea, facial edema, weakness, heart irregularities
Epirubicin	Hair loss, loss of menses, anemia, leukopenia, bone marrow depression, esophagitis, infections, nausea, vomiting, inflamed oral cavity, discolored urine, abscess, diarrhea, GI tract ulcers, skin reddening, inflammation of veins and clots, tissue necrosis or degeneration , kidney disorders, hot flashes
Cytoxan	Abdominal pain and cramps, hair loss, infections, irregular menses, leukopenia, skin and nails darkening, nausea, vomiting skin blisters and thickening, fatigue, pericarditis, low platelets, kidney and liver toxicities, shortness of breath, high blood glucose, hives, skin rashes and itching, inflamed oral cavity
Taxol Plant Akaloid	Allergic reactions, skin rashes and reddening, hair loss, anemia, leukopenia, joint pain, diarrhea, nausea, vomiting, shortness of breath, weakness, fatigue, nerve damage, liver toxicity, hypotension, abscess, inflamed veins and mouth
Femara - Al	Abdominal pain and cramps, hair loss, anxiety, depression, joint pain, constipation, diarrhea, drowsiness, shortness of breath, fatigue, weakness, insomnia, sweating, headaches, limb and muscle pain, high blood pressure, itching, nausea, vomiting, weight gain, skin rashes, abnormal liver functions, blurred vision, long menses, bone loss, blot clotting disorders, urinary tract infections
Evista	cloudy or cloudy urine, chest pain, burning on urination, infection, body aches, infection, body aches and pains, runny nose, cough, congestion, dry throat, loss of voice, leg cramps, skin rash, swelling of hands and feet, vaginal itching
Tamoxifen - SER	Bone pain, nausea and vomiting, black stools, bloody urine, dry skin, itching, confusion, decrease urine, hot flashes, profuse sweating, weight gain, loosening of skin and mucous membranes, leg swelling, cough, dizziness, fast heartbeat

Docetaxel	Swelling of abdomen, face, fingers, hands, feet, and lower legs, weight gain, fatigue and weakness, red scaly skin, low or high blood pressure, fainting and dizziness and headaches
Trastuzumab (Herceptin)	Dizziness, fever and/or chills, headaches, nausea, vomiting, shortness of breath, skin rash, allergic reactions, weakness, cardiotoxicity
Bevacizumab (Avastin)	Hypertension, protein in the urine, decreased nerve sensation, heart dysfunction, perforations of the stomach and intestines
Vinorelbine	Hair loss, anemia, constipation, fatigue, weakness, leukopenia, nausea, vomiting, numbness, inflamed veins, loss of appetite, joint, chest and muscle pain, inflamed oral cavity, loss of bowel motility, low platelets
Gemzar	Constipation, diarrhea, malaise, loss of appetite, nausea, vomiting, muscle pain, runny noise, sweating, insomnia
Procrit (Erythropoietin)	Fever, diarrhea, nausea, vomiting, swelling weakness, fatigue, shortness of breath, upper respiratory infection, dizziness, trunk and bone pain, headaches
Neupogen (GSF) Granulocyte colony stimulating factor	Nausea and vomiting, bone pain, hair loss, diarrhea, constipation, fever, inflamed mouth, fatigue, loss of appetite, shortness of breath, headaches, cough, skin rash, chest pain

ADJUVANT HORMONAL THERAPY

Adjuvants treatments are treatments needed in addition to the primary surgical treatment and radiation treatment. Systemic adjuvant therapy, may be chemotherapy drugs, anti-estrogen therapy, and targeted therapies. Systemic therapy and radiation therapy is indicated to prevent or delay the progression of metastatic disease, tumor spread, and disease recurrence in order to prolong of the life of a patient with breast cancer. The current thought about early staged breast cancer (invasive breast cancers up to 1 cm in size) is that many patients will have distant micrometastases or small foci of tumor spread to distant sites that will in time progress to metastatic disease.

Current chemotherapy in patients with 1 to 3 positive lymph nodes consists of treating the patient systemically with the administration of Cyclophosphamide, Doxorubicin and a taxane, Paclitaxel or Docetaxel.

Patients with lymph node positive disease or tumor metastatic to lymph nodes benefit from the use of taxanes.

The response of breast tissue to hormones has been known for a long time. The treatment for patients with breast cancer is dependent on the hormonal status of the tumor, whether or not the tumor is estrogen (ER) and progesterone receptor (PR) positive or negative. These prognostically significant tumor markers are determined directly on a section of tumor which is mounted directly on glass slides, prepared and specially stained and examined microscopically by the pathologist in order to determine the presence or absence of the ER and PR receptors. The results and status of the ER and PR receptors are usually included as part of the surgical pathology report. [22]

These hormone receptors should be determined on all invasive breast cancers so that the oncologist can appropriately treat patients who have hormonally responsive tumors. About 70% of breast cancers have positive estrogen receptors (ER) and 60% are positive for progesterone receptor (PR). The positivity of the receptors increases with the age of the patient. Approximately 30% of breast cancer tumors are ER-negative and about 8% of these ER-negative tumors will respond to hormonal ablative therapy. Breast cancers that are ER-positive tend to recur or relapse after many years. Breast cancers that are ER-negative tend to relapse or recur earlier than ER-positive tumors.[23]

Breast cancers are categorized into the following types on the basis of hormonal assessment. See next table.

Table 21-4.

Receptor Type	Percentage	Response Hormone Rx
ER +, PR +	65	70%
ER +, PR -	10	33%
ER - , PR +	5	33%
ER - , PR - or Unknown	25	Treatment usually not effective

ER+, PR+ tumors are usually low grade tumors and of a better prognosis and are clinically more likely to respond to adjuvant endocrine therapy (anti-hormonal therapy).

ER+, PR+ tumors have a 70% response rate to anti-hormonal therapy. Up to 33% of **ER+, PR- and ER-, PR+** tumors respond to anti-hormonal therapy. **ER-, PR-** tumors of unknown status usually do not respond to anti-hormonal therapy.

Adjuvant endocrine therapy (anti-hormonal therapy) is treatment for women with hormone receptor-positive breast cancer which is usually taken for 5 years. Women who are premenopausal or perimenopausal and male breast cancer should be treated with Tamoxifen for 5 years. The major drugs used have been **Tamoxifen and Raloxifene which are selective estrogen receptor modulators (SERMs).** Patients who progress on initial anti-hormonal therapy usually also respond favorably to second, third and fourth generation drugs for treatment. However, the class of drugs that shut down the production of estrogen, the **aromatase inhibitors (AIs),** i.e. Anastrozole, Letrozole and Exemestane are becoming the preferred endocrine therapy. For postmenopausal women with ER+ breast cancers an AI should be given for five years or for 2 to 3 years then followed by Tamoxifen for 2 years. Women who were started on Tamoxifen for 2 to 3 years can be switched to an AI. Fulvestrant is the single member of a new drug class called the **selective estrogen receptor downregulator (SERD)** that down regulate estrogen and progesterone. [24]

Whatever, adjuvant endocrine therapy is selected is a decision which must be made between patient and doctor. There is always a risk for tumor recurrence in women with breast cancer. Residual or microscopic disease may be present and must be treated. Even if you have no evidence of disease in your lymph nodes you may be at increased risk for recurrence and you should discuss this with your physician. Ask about your risk and whether or not there are any additional tests that can be done to determine whether or not you need additional treatment.

Women who are low risk for recurrence or without advanced disease or who have low grade breast cancers are treated by surgical excision, with or without radiation and an anti-estrogen. Not all patients who are ER-positive respond to anti-estrogen.

It is known that women who have been previously treated for breast cancer are still at risk for developing recurrent cancer. Up to 60% of patients with tumors that are ER-negative have recurrences of disease. Current adjuvant therapy recommendations are ovarian ablation (surgical removal of the ovaries or irradiation or drug treatment) and/or Tamoxifen and systemic treatment by chemotherapy. The standard use of Tamoxifen for ER/PR receptor positive tumors has been shown to reduce the risk of recurrence of disease and increase the survival rate for patients. [25] The Early Breast Cancer Trials Collaborative Group in 1998 demonstrated this outcome in over 36,000 patients receiving Tamoxifen for at least five years and beyond. [26]

The third generation **aromatase inhibitors(AIs)** are **Anastrazole, Exemestane, Letrazole, Raloxifene, and Femara**. The aromatase inhibitors (AIs) are mixed estrogen antagonists and agonists. They effectively block estrogen and reduce the risk of breast cancer recurrence. They prevent the conversion of the hormones androstenedione and testosterone to estrogen and decrease the circulating estrogen hormonal level. Tamoxifen does not have such properties and this is why endometrial hyperplasia and vaginal bleeding may occur along with other toxicities, including thromboembolic or clotting diseases like pulmonary emboli (blood clots to the lung), and deep vein thrombosis (blood clots in the legs and other sites) and bone loss.

Studies have been conducted looking at the effects that second-, third- and fourth-generation AIs had on bone loss. There is some evidence that the AI drug, Exemestane which has a structure like male hormone, androgen has less impact on bone turnover and bone loss and is protective of bone. The AI Letrozole, however, appears to be associated with increase bone turnover and bone loss.

The AIs were first evaluated in patients with advanced metastatic disease. The AI's become second line therapy for patients who have failed to respond to tamoxifen therapy. For a postmenopausal woman with an estrogen receptor positive breast cancer, it is recommended that an AI be used as either initial therapy or after treatment with Tamoxifen. The AI, Anastrozole has shown a longer disease free intervals and increased time to disease recurrence than Tamoxifen.[27,28] Patients taking Anastrazole also experience less hot flashes, vaginal bleeding and discharge, deep vein thrombosis or clots, strokes and endometrial cancer, but are more likely to experience bone fractures. The good news is that we now have treatment to offer women whose tumors progress on prior anti-hormonal therapy as second chance where they can be expected to respond to second-, third- and fourth-line treatments.

The use of anti-estrogens has been found to beneficial in both premenopausal and postmenopausal patients with ER receptor positive tumors, showing a risk reduction of tumor recurrence by 50%. Patients with lymph node positive disease have a risk reduction for recurrence by 43%. Patients that have large operable tumors should be given neoadjuvant therapy or treatment before surgery to reduce the size of the tumor and thereby enable the patient to undergo breast-conserving surgery instead of complete breast removal or mastectomy.

It is important to shut down estrogen production completely in younger women. Ovarian ablation by either surgical removal of the ovaries or irradiation of the ovaries, benefits young premenopausal women with lymph node metastases. [29] There are also drugs available that have an effect like luteinizing hormone releasing hormone (LHRH), a hormone in the pituitary gland of the brain which shuts down the ovaries ability to produce estrogen. Besides these drugs, anti-estrogen agents like Tamoxifen or Exemestane should be given.

Breast cancers are classified as Estrogen and Progesterone receptor positive or negative (ER+/- and PR+/-) and can also be further subclassified based on HER2 status. HER2 is also another diagnostic test and prognostic marker of breast tumors. HER2 is an oncogene, p185, a tumor gene that encodes a protein, belonging to the family of epidermal growth factor receptors (EGRF). The HER2 receptor promotes increased cellular division and growth of the tumor. HER2 positive tumors have a high nuclear grade and the patient survival rate is usually shorter. The HER2 or HercepTest is performed directly on breast tumor by either immunohistochemistry (IHC) or by FISH. The HER2 test is performed routinely on all breast cancers and is reported as HER2 overexpression (positive) or HER2 negative. If the test is performed by IHC and has a borderline or 1+ result, the test is usually repeated by FISH. Breast tumors that are HER2+ or display HER2 overexpression are usually clinically more aggressive than HER2- negative tumors. The HER2 test is a good predictor of whether or not a patient is likely to respond to the targeted therapy drug Herceptin (Trastuzumab). For HER2+ patients and patients with advanced disease or metastatic tumor the drug Trastuzumab has now become standard treatment. [30,31] **Trastuzumab** is a monoclonal antibody that targets the epidermal growth factor or HER2 receptor. Patients with HER2+ breast tumors who receive adjuvant Trastuzumab have been found to have a lower the risk of cancer recurrence by 58%. [12,13] Evidence suggests that the addition of a taxane also benefits patient with HER2+ breast cancers.

HER2 has been an excellent biomarker targeting tumors that overexpress HER2, but we realize in the last 10 years that half of the women with HER2 + breast cancers do not benefit from treatment with Trastuzumab and are resistant to such therapy. New biomarkers must be discovered for HER2+ tumors and we must stir the interest of pharmaceutical companies to develop drugs for patients based on newly discovered biomarkers to help patients that do not benefit from Trastuzumab treatment.

It was hoped that the controversial drug **Avastin (Bevacizumab)** which is a monoclonal antibody would benefit breast cancer patients. The monoclonal antibody, Bevacizumab destroys the blood supply of tumors by inhibiting vascular endothelial growth factor (VEGF), a factor that promotes the growth of cells lining and forming new blood vessels to supply blood to the tumor. Bevacizumab has been used in the treatment of colon and rectal cancer and lung cancer. [28] The drug when used with Taxol in one study showed slow the progression of tumor growth, but not significantly enough to prolong patient survival. When Avastin was added to Taxotere in treating women with advanced breast cancer the progression-free survival was increased by two months, a 23% improvement. However, these findings were not duplicated in more recent studies which indicated the Avastin is not beneficial in the treatment of breast cancer patients. Avastin has neither increased the progression free-survival nor the overall survival of patients. Patients who received Avastin (Bevacizumab) and Paclitaxel were no better off than patients who received Paclitaxel alone. It is recommended that Avastin (Bevacizumab) no longer be given to breast cancer patients with HER2 + breast tumors.

Molecular diagnostics by ER, PR and HER2 has allowed for the further classification of breast cancers into the following subtypes;

Table 21-5.

Subtypes
ER +, PR +, HER2 -
ER +, PR +, HER2 +
ER -, PR -, HER2 – (Triple Negative Cancer)
ER -, PR -, HER2 overexpressing

Triple Negative Breast Cancer (TNBC)

Triple negative breast cancers are ER-, PR-, HER2- tumors. These tumors are aggressive. Patients with TNBC have a higher rate of tumor growth and larger size tumors. They also have an increased number of axillary lymph nodes that contain metastatic tumor. These patients tend to be younger women, African-American women and women with the BRCA-1 mutated cancers. TNBC is treated with radiation therapy, surgery and chemotherapy. TNBC does not respond to hormonal therapy or Herceptin (Trastuzumab). Patients with triple negative breast cancer , TNBC usually show an earlier recurrence of disease [33] and poor survival after recurrence. These tumors usually have different routes of metastatic spread or the cancer when compared to other breast cancers. A study by Lin showed that 14% of patients had central nervous system (CNS) or brain involvement at the time of the initial relapse or recurrence and 46% of patients had CNS or metastases (cancer spread to the brain) before death. These patients were also 4 times more likely to have spread to vital organs like the lungs and liver within 5 years than patients with other types of breast cancer.[34]

The prognosis for these patients with TNBC is usually poor compared to other subtypes of breast cancer.[35] Recently an mRNA for growth hormone releasing hormone (GHRH) receptor was found in a human triple-negative breast cancer cell line grown in a laboratory. Studies have demonstrated that targeting this receptor may be an option for treatment of these tumors. [36] **Gemfitinib**, an epidermal Growth Factor Receptor inhibitor, may also be a prospective treatment for these tumors in the future. Poly-ADP-ribose polymerase **(PARP)**-inhibitors, an enzyme that is necessary for the repair of the DNA in a cell could be inhibited by new drugs targeting the enzyme, this when combined with other chemotherapy drugs could possibly result in effective treatment for TNBC.[37] Hopefully, researchers may develop other forms of targeted therapy drugs that may be capable of changing the gene expression of tumor cells so that they behave in a more normal manner and be sensitized to regular breast cancer therapies.

TARGETED THERAPY FOR BREAST CANCER TREATMENT
HOPE FOR THE FUTURE

Hormonal therapy has allowed researchers to look at ways to reverse the progression of breast cancer based upon the presence of the ER receptor positivity. The ER receptor is a target. Molecular biology has allowed us to look more closely at patients who do not express ER receptor positivity and also to look at their lack of clinical response to hormonal therapy. It has allowed us to look at the biologic processes and identify more targets such as the Human Epidermal Growth Factor Receptor- 2 (HER2) and the epidermal growth factor receptor (EGFR), which have become new therapeutic targets for targeted therapy. HER2 triggers pathways within the cell associated with an enzyme, tyrosinase kinase that results in increased proliferation of cells that are resistant to cellular death, and the proliferation or increased growth of blood vessels or angiogenesis. HER2 overexpression occurs in 25-30% of breast cancers. Studies done in mice using a monoclonal (single clone) antibody to HER2 showed that breast cancers with HER2 when exposed to the monoclonal antibody to HER2 have demonstrated inhibition of tumor growth. [38,39]. This led to the development of the anti-HER2 antibody, Trastuzumab. Trastuzumab's effectiveness has been established for patients with HER2 overexpression. Multiple studies using Trastuzumab alone and in combination with other chemotherapeutic drugs have been done to see whether or not the drugs would have an antagonistic or synergistic effect on breast tumors, in other words whether or not the drug combinations would impede the tumor growth when used with Trastuzumab.[40] Chemotherapy when given with Trastuzumab has been found to be associated with a better long-term survival than Trastuzumab followed by chemotherapy.[41] The combination of Trastuzumab with the drug Vinorelbine has resulted in a 75% overall reduction in breast cancer recurrence. Patients receiving Trastuzumab with Paclitaxel (Taxol) and Carboplatin showed progression of the disease. [42]

Trastuzumab is the first generation targeted therapy for HER2-positive breast cancer. Not all patients benefit from the therapy with Trastuzumab, some develop resistance. The new targeted agent Everolimus (Affnitor) in a recent clinical trial of women with metastatic HER2 overexpressing breast cancer 35% of the 47 patients achieved a partial response or stabilization of their disease. [43] Additional new second generation drugs are being developed and studied to ensure that patients that become resistant the other therapies will have the benefit of other promising therapies.

Anti-EGFR

Epithelial Growth Factor (EGFR) is expressed by up to 36% of breast tumors and conceivably may be a good target for therapy. C225 has been found to inhibit EGFR and the proliferation of cells. It has been investigated in some lung cancers and colorectal cancer, but has not been investigated in breast cancer. Other monoclonal antibodies have been developed that target EGFR include ABX-EGF, EMD 7200 and h-R3. ZD183 has antineoplastic activity in several cancers, including breast cancer. It causes increased fragmentation of DNA. [44] Phase 2 trials are being conducted with ZD183 and hormonal therapy in ER receptor positive patients.

OSI-774 has demonstrated strong antitumor activity against cancer cells that express EGFR. CI-1033 has activity against cancer cells that overexpress EGFR, which is detected at a high level in many breast cancers. Trial studies as a single agent and with Anthracycline, Taxane and Capecitabine and with Trastuzumab are being conducted. CI-1033 irreversibly inhibits signaling of the erbB family and has evidence of effectiveness against breast cancer cells and may work together with Cisplatin. Tyrosine kinase inhibitors also fall under the category of anti-

EGFR therapy. **Lapatinib (Tykerb)** is a dual kinase inhibitor of HER2 and EGFR. It is a combination of Lapatinib and Trastuzumab and is emerging as a new treatment option for patients receiving chemotherapy and Trastuzumab.[45, 46] The FDA approved Lapatinib in combination with capecitabine for the treatment of HER2 + advanced breast cancer that has progressed after treatment with Trastuzumab in 2007.

Anti-Angiogenesis Therapy

The formation of new blood vessels, angiogenesis causes a tumor to be nourished and enables it to grow and spread and invade other tissues. Inhibitors of angiogenesis that thwart the signaling of **vascular endothelial growth factor (VEGF)** in early stage breast cancer have been discovered. The monoclonal antibody **Bevacizumab** is an antibody directed against VEGF and has been found to inhibit the growth of human tumors. A phase 2 trial showed an objective response in 17% of patients previously treated for metastatic breast carcinoma[47] Other VEFG targeted drugs being studied are **sunitinib, sorafenib, and AZD2171.**[48]

Matrix metalloproteinase (MMP) inhibitors may cause the spread of tumor by destroying the basement membrane of ducts giving tumor cells access to surrounding tissue. Clinical trials have been disappointing however, because of adverse reactions. CD-527, 632 another agent which inhibits VEGF also inhibit tumor growth and is tolerated well with no significant toxicity. Angiozyme, a ribosome cleaves the messenger RNA for certain receptor proteins and destroys certain protein products is being studied. Vitaxin, an antibody to alphaVbeta 3 has antiangiogenic activity. Other inhibitors being studied are RGD-containing peptides and endostatin, a natural inhibitor with antiangiogenic activity which induces cell death. ZD6126 potentiates radiation-mediated anti-tumor effects.

The future of the treatment of breast cancer is becoming brighter as new antibodies are developed and targeted to EGFR and various pathways that inhibit the growth of tumor cells and blood vessels and block receptor sites. This may eventually hold the cure to this dreaded disease and other cancers as well. Although breast cancers are similar, they are all different. Breast cancers need to be separated into subgroups with therapies that are tailored for the treatment of the particular groups. New approaches will be developed as new agents are studied. Breast cancer may soon become a treatable chronic condition or may one day be completely erradicated.

References:

1. Photographs. White Fish Mitosis. Cell Division Genetic consequences, ttp://biog10104.bio.Cornell.edu/BioG101_104/tutorials/cell_divisi on/wf_review_fs.html2.
2. Fisher, Kathleen. The Natural Science 412A/B/C Course. Drawings. Http://www.biologylessons.sdsu.edu/ta/classes/lab8/index.html.
3. Greenbay PA, Hortobagyi GN, Smith TL, et al. Long-term follow-up of patients with complete remission following combination therapy for metastatic breast cancer. J Clin Oncology 1996; 14:2197-2205. Abstract
4. Hayes, D. Is there a standard type and duration of adjuvant chemotherapy? Breast 2009; 18 (Suppl.1): S15 (Abstr S37).
5. Citron ML, Berry DA, Cirrincione C, et al. Randomized trial of dose- dense versus conventionally scheduled and sequential versus concurrent combination chemotherapy as postoperative adjuvant treatment of node positive primary breast cancer first report of intergroup trial C9741/Cancer and Leukemia Group B Trial 9741.
6. Ellis M "Taxane-based chemotherapy for node-positive breast cancer -- Take-home lessons" *N Engl J Med* 2010; 362: 2122-24.
7. Sparano JA, et al Weekly paclitaxel in the adjuvant treatment of breast cancer, NEJM 2008; 3581663-1671.
8. Gradishar,William,J,BreninChristiana,Anderson,ME.Chemothera-peutic Options for early and late stage breast cancer.
9. Cleator, S.; Tsimelzon A., et al.Gene expression patterns for Doxorubicin and Cyclophosamide response and resistance Breast Cancer Res Treat. 206; 95(3)229-33.
10. Praga C., Bergh J., et al. Risk of acute myeloid leukemia and myelodysplastic syndrome in trials of adjuvant Epirubicin for early breast cancer correlation with doses of Epirubicin and

Cyclophosamide, J Clin Oncology 2005; 23(18)4179-91.

11. Thomson Healthcare, Micromedex. 2006.

12. Chusteka, Z and Lie, D., Medscape article 533999. American Society of Clinical Oncology 2006 Annual Meeting, AMA early release article JAMA June 2005.

13. Piccart, MJ. Trastuzumab in the adjuvant setting an expert interview. Medscape Hematology Oncology 2006, 9(1) article *520064.*

14. Rossari, J., et al "Bevacizumab combined with chemotherapy as first-line treatment of metastatic breast cancer patients: a meta-analysis based on studies having randomized 2,695 patients" *EBCC* 2010; Abstract122.

15. Seidman, A., The Evolving Role of Gemcitabine in the Management of Metastatic Breast Cancer. MedPoint Office of medical Education, 2003.

16. Barclay, L. et Lie, D. , Swain. Letrazole may be useful adjuvant therapy for endocrine responsive breast cancer. NEJM 2005; 353:2747-2757. 2807-2809.

17. Lie, Desiree et Barclay, L. Letrazole may be useful adjuvant for endocrine-responsive breast cancer. Medscape article 520760. Jan 2006.

18. Thomson Micromedex, Docetaxel., Thomson Healthcare. 2006.

19. Procrit Full Prescribing Information. Amgen, Inc. 2000.

20. Bronchud, MH et al. The use of granulocyte colony-stimulating factor to increase the intensity of treatment with Doxorubicin in patients with advanced breast and ovarian cancer. Br. J. Cancer. 1989,60:121-128.

21.Barclay, L et Lie, D., Trastuzumab may prompt change in practice recommendations for Her2-Positive breast cancer, Medscape CME News. Oct 19, 2005. Reference to New Engl Journal of Medicine 2005; 3531659-1684, 1734-1736. References:

23.Goldhirsch A, Wood WC, Gelber, RD, et al. Meeting highlights updated international expert consensus on the primary therapy of early breast cancer. J Clin Oncol. 2003; 21:3357-3365.

24. Mullan, PB, Millikan RC. Molecular subtyping of breast cancer:

opportunities for new therapeutic approaches. *Cell Mol Life Sci.* 2007;64(24):3219-3232.

24. Jones, Stephen E. Update in Hormonal Therapy A 2004 Perspective. Physicians Education Resource. 2004.

25. Alberg, AJ, Lam AP, et al. Epidemiology, prevention and early detection of breast cancer. Curr Opin Oncol. 199,11:435-441.

26. Tamoxifen for early breast cancer an overview of the randomized trials. Early Breast Cancer Trialists' Collaborative   Group. Lancet. 1998, 351:1451-1467.

27. The ATAC Trialists' Group. Anastrozole alone or in combination with tamoxifen versus tamoxifen alone for adjuvant treatment of postmenopausal women with early-stage breast cancer. Cancer. 2003, 98:1802-1810.

28. FDA News PO4-23, February 1,2007. http://www.fda.gov/CDER/DRUG/infopage/avastin/avastinQ&A.htm

29. Ovarian ablation in early breast cancer overview of the randomized trials. Early Breast Cancer Trialists' Collaborative Group. Lancet. 1996; 348:118

30. Piccart-Gebhart MJ, Procter M, Leyland-Jones, B. et al. Trastuzumab after adjuvant chemotherapy in Her2-positive breast cancer. N. Eng J Med. 2005; 353:1659-1672 Abstract.31. Tripathy, Debu. Advances in Treatment of Her2-Positive Early Breast Cancer. Expert Interview. Medscape Hematology-Oncology. 2006; 9(1). 2/28/2006.

31. Romond, EH, Perez EA, Bryant J, et al. Trastuzumab plus adjuvant chemotherapy for operable Her2-positive breast cancer. N Engl J Med 2005; 353:1673-1684. Abstract

32. Joensuu, H, Kellokump-Lehtinen, PL, Bono P, et al. Trastuzumab in combination with Docetaxel or vinorelbine as adjuvant treatment of breast cancer the FinHer trial. Breast Cancer Res Treat. 2005, 94(suppl 1)S5. Abstract 2

33. Koster, Frank, Engel J.B. Et al., Triple Negative Recurrence Hazard, Medwire, June 4, 2008

34. Yin, Wen-Jin, Jin, Song Lu, et al. Prognosis of Women with Triple Negative Breast Cancers. MedWire Online June 10, 2008.

35. Heitz, F, Harter P, Traut, A, et al. Cerebral metastases (CM) in

breast cancer (BC) with focus on triple-negative tumors. *J ClinOncol* [2008 ASCO Annual Meeting Proceedings (Post-Meeting Edition)]. 2008;26(15S):1010.

36. Dent, Rebecca, Hanna, WM, et al., Triple-Negative Breast cancer Growth hormone-releasing hormone,GHRH antagonist. MedWire July 16, 2008.
37. Tutt, A "Early phase proof of concept studies and rationale for patient selection" *IMPAKT* 2010; Abstract 5IN.
38. Carey, LA, Rugo, HS, Marcom PK, et al. TBCRC 001: EGFR inhibition with cetuximab added to carboplatin in metastatic triple-negative breast cancer. Proc Am Soc Clin Oncol. 2008;26:43s. Abstract 1009
39. Drebin JA, Link VC, Greene MI. Monoclonal antibodies specific for the neu oncogene product directly mediate anti-tumor effects in vivo. Oncogene. 1988, 2:387-394.
40. Hudziak, RM, Lewis, GD, Winget, M, et al. The p185HER2 monoclonal antibody has antiproliferative effects in vitro and sensitizes human breast tumor cells to tumor necrosis factor. Mol Cell Biol. 1989; 9:1165-1172.
42. Burstein HJ, Kuter, I, Campos, SM, et al. Clinical activity of Trastuzumab and vinorelbine in women with HER2-overexpressing metastatic breast cancer. J Clin Oncol. 2001,19:2722-2730.
43. American Society for Clinical Oncology (ASCO) 2008 annual meeting. Targeted Therapy for Breast Cancer.
44. Morrow P.K. et al, "Phase I/II trial of Everolimus (RAD001) and Trastuzumab in patients with Trastuzumab-resistant, HER2-overexpressing breast cancer" *J Clin Oncol* 2010; 28: Abstract 1014.
45. Meden, H, Beneke, A, Hesse. T, et al. Weekly intravenous recombinant humanized anti-P185HER2 monoclonal antibody (Herceptin) plus docetaxel in patients with metastatic breast cancer pilot study. Anticancer Res. 2001,21:1301-1305.
46. Bontenbal, M, Seynaeve, C, Stouthard, J, et al. Randomized study comparing efficacy / toxicity of monotherapy Trastuzumab followed by monotherapy docetaxel at progression, and

combination Trastuzumab/docetaxel as first line chemotherapy in HER2-neu positive metastatic breast cancer (HERTAX study). Proc Am Soc Clin Oncol. 2008;26:44s. Abstract 1014.

47. O'Shaugnessy, J, Blackwell, K, Burstein, HJ, et al. A randomized study of lapatinib alone or in combination with trastuzumab in heavily pretreated HER2+ metastatic breast cancer progressing on trastuzumab therapy. Proc Am Soc Clin Oncol. 2008;26:44s. Abstract 1015.

48. Normanno N, Campiglio M, De LA, et al. Cooperative inhibitory effect of ZD183(Iressa) in combination with trastuzumab (Herceptin) on human breast cancer cell growth. Ann Oncol. 2002,13:65-72.

49. Sledge G, Miller K, Novotny W, et al. Phase II trial of single agent rhuMab VEGF in patients with relapsed metastatic breast cancer. Program and abstracts of the 36th Annual Meeting of the American Society of Clinical Oncology; May 20-23, 2000; San Francisco, California. Abstract 5C.

Lessons To Be Learned

1) If your physician states that you need chemotherapy you should ask your physician how far the cancer has spread.
2) Ask your physician what type of breast cancer you have.
3) Know the ER, PR and Her2 receptor status of the cancer.
4) Ask your physician what are your chances for a cure.
5) Ask whether or not you are a candidate for chemotherapy before surgery.
6) Ask your physician what type of chemotherapy drugs you will be on and what type of side effects can be expected.
7) Ask your physician what you should do if you experience any side effects and who you should contact if you have an emergency or any questions.
8) Ask your physician if your tumor can be treated with Tamoxifen or another anti-estrogen.
9) Let your physician if you have a history of blood clots or a family history of clotting disorders.
10) Ask your physician which anti-estrogen is better for you.

11) Ask your physician if you should take drugs to suppress your ovaries or whether or not surgical removal or chemical suppression of your ovaries is warranted.

RADIATION THERAPY

Most patients undergoing breast-conserving surgery, receive radiation treatments to lower the risk for local-regional recurrence. Women who have had mastectomies have a risk for recurrence should also receive radiation treatment. Patients with Ductal Carcinoma in situ (DCIS) and who may be considered high risk for cancer recurrence may also benefit from radiation. Many patients are given radiation to the entire breast, but there are radiation treatment centers that are using limited-field radiation therapy that targets the radiation to a specific area of the breast adjacent to the tumor site. This is exceedingly advantageous, since it reduces the risk of long-term side effects of radiation and limits the amount of normal cells, which are exposed to the radiation.

Patients that have had chemotherapy need radiation also. Radiotherapy is necessary in order to attain adequate local tumor control. It is not useful against cancer that has already spread to distant parts of the body. Chemotherapy does not provide local control. It provides systemic control or control over the entire body. Residual tumor cells may be present in the breast can cause recurrence. These residual tumor cells must be treated to limit the chance of recurrence. The goal of radiation is to cure or shrink the early stage cancer. Ten years after receiving radiation treatment, a recent study showed that 95% of postmenopausal patients with early stage were found to be from recurrence of their breast cancer. Radiation treatments are effective and very few patients undergoing radiation experience lethal side effects and few experience minor side effects.

The types of radiation therapy are: pre-operative, adjuvant and prophylactic. If radiation is done before surgery it is called pre-operative therapy. If it is done after surgery it is called adjuvant therapy. If an area is treated even though CT scans and MRI scans are negative, it is called prophylactic radiation. When surgery, chemotherapy and radiation are used, the treatment plan is coordinated and devised by the surgeon, the medical oncologist and the radiation oncologist.

The radiation treatment team usually consists of a radiation oncologist (a physician trained to treat patients with cancer), a radiation physicist (a person who ensures that the right radiation dose is received), a radiation therapist or technologist (the operator of the equipment for the treatment) and a radiation therapy nurse, who may follow up with the patient during treatment and deal with any questions and the side effects of the treatment.

How Radiation Works

Radiation is essentially energy waves or particles that can alter DNA and molecules which control the life cycle of the cell. Radiation acts on actively dividing cells and is less effective on cells in the resting G_0 phase. It is similar to chemotherapy in that it cannot distinguish between normal and abnormal cells, so damage is done to normal and abnormal cells. The damage done is part of the side effects or the therapy.

There are two types of ionizing radiation used for cancer treatment:
- photons (x-rays and gamma rays)
- particles (electrons, protons, neutrons, alpha particles and beta particles)

Radiation in cancer treatment uses high-energy x-rays or other types of radiation to kill cancer cells. The delivery method varies according to the place and type of cancer. External radiation uses a machine to deliver the radiation to the tumor. Internal radiation uses radioactive wires, needles, seeds or catheters to deliver the radiation directly to or near the tumor site.

In a study by Dr. Jagsi [1] 8% to 14% of 281 patients who had a mastectomy with axillary lymph nodes resection and no evidence of tumor in the lymph nodes developed local and regional recurrence and metastases. [2] Microscopic cancer at the surgical margins has been found to be a significant factor in the recurrence rate of cancer. All Stage II node negative patients should be offered postoperative irradiation to reduce the risk of recurrence of tumor.

Radiation Therapy After Lumpectomy

Patients diagnosed with ductal carcinoma in situ may have subsequent local recurrences similarly to recurrences as in invasive ductal carcinoma. Mastectomy alone cured 95% of ductal carcinoma in situ patients in the past. The present trend however, is breast conservation and to offer lumpectomy with radiation in both ductal carcinoma in situ and invasive carcinoma. Follow-up has shown after 90 months that recurrence of invasive disease decreased from 13% to 40% and recurrence of DCIS decreased from 13% to 80% with the addition of radiation therapy. [3]

The contraindications to breast conservation therapy are:
- Multiple primary breast tumors in different quadrants of the breast
- Diffuse mammographic microcalcifications
- Previous history of radiation to the breast
- Patient unable to lie flat or grasp and move their arm
- Tumor in a breast of small size
- Autoimmune or collagen vascular disease
- Obesity with markedly enlarged breasts.

New radiation techniques like targeted treatment are being tried in some centers on obese women to avoid the radiation of surrounding normal tissue to improve the cosmetic outcome. [4, 5]

First and second trimester **pregnancy** was considered a contraindication to breast conservation therapy, but a recent study by Dr. Theribault at the University of Texas M.D. Anderson Cancer Center in Houston tracking some 57 pregnant women who were diagnosed with breast cancer has shown that cancer treatment in pregnancy is not a grim diagnosis. Breast cancer in pregnant women can be treated successfully with delivery of healthy babies. Termination of the pregnancy is not required. Most of the patients in the study had advanced disease at the time of diagnosis and mastectomy was the surgical treatment of choice. Radiation when needed can be postponed until the birth of the infant and chemotherapy has been given to some patients up to three weeks prior to delivery. [6]

When **internal radiation** is used a balloon is placed in the lumpectomy cavity to treat the tissue surrounding the cavity that is left after the breast tissue has been removed. A single source of radiation is delivered with 2 treatments being given for 5 days and lessening the total treatment time. This method however, currently is not recommended for all patients. High dose radiation brachytherapy (**HDR brachytherapy**) uses catheters that are implanted near the lumpectomy surgical site. High doses of radiation are given to the site without affecting the surrounding tissue and reducing the need for a mastectomy or external radiation. Both methods are effective options for treatment and can be discussed with your radiation oncologist to determine if these methods of treatment are suitable options for your treatment plan.

External radiation by Tomo-therapy(3-dimensional radiotherapy), directs beams of radiation directly to the tumor. Treatment coordinates are adjusted to limit or avoid damage to muscle, the spine, lungs and heart. Conventional external radiation directs the beams of radiation in a few directions whereas, Tomo-therapy delivers more precise heavy doses of radiation from 360 ^{0} and is an option in some centers. Mayo Clinic in Arizona has reduced the number of weeks of therapy to four weeks by using the Mobetron to deliver intraoperative (during surgery) external radiation therapy. The University College of London's large clinical trial of **targeted intraoperative radiotherapy (TARGIT)**, found the use intraoperative low energy x-rays in the tumor bed for 20 to 35 minutes was not inferior to standard conventional radiation treatment plan that lasts 5 to 6 weeks. This treatment is still experimental. It is hoped that this accelerated partial breast irradiation which can be completed in 1 to 2 days may become the standard of treatment in the future. [7]

Do not be afraid to ask your radiation oncologist any questions that you may have about your treatment. The radiation oncologist will usually tell you what type of treatment is recommended in your case, how many treatments you will receive, when the treatments will start, when the treatments will end, the length of the treatments, the risks and side effects of the treatment and whom you should contact if you experience any side effects. Your radiation oncologist will also be able to tell you the cosmetic effects of the treatment, how your breast will look and feel and how you should take care of your skin during the treatment. If you have any questions at all including as to why you need the treatment and what will happen if you don't take the treatment, you should ask the radiation oncologist those questions. There is no such thing as a dumb question when it come to your health and your quality of life.

If you are having conventional radiation treatments, the sessions are usually Monday through Friday. Each treatment will be short. However, your first visit to the radiation center after surgical removal of a breast mass (lumpectomy) may take a few hours. Additional

X-rays will be taken with a CT scan of the chest and coordinates set to plan the three dimensional treatment. Your radiation oncologist will plan your treatment based on the physical examination, mammograms, CT scan, other X-rays, land the laboratory and pathology reports.

After the treatment has been planned the radiation therapist may prepare a body cast that perfectly matches your upper torso so that you will be in the same position for each treatment. Your chest will be marked and later tattooed using a small needlepoint pricks with dark dye. These marks correspond with the area being treated. This area is based on your predetermined coordinates to make sure that the least amount of normal tissue will be exposed to radiation. These coordinates will be used to place you in the proper position on the treatment table for succeeding treatments.

Radiation after Mastectomy

Radiation therapy is used after mastectomy for tumors larger than 2.5 cm and when cancer is found in lymph nodes in the axilla (under the arm) or near the ribs. Early Stage I and II (T1-2 N1) breast cancer is usually treated with surgery followed by radiation. Radiation increases the overall survival of Stage I and II breast cancer patients from 43% to 87% and the recurrence free five year survival to 83%. The major adverse effects of radiotherapy are radiation pneumonitis (inflammation of the lungs) and the development of pericardial effusion or fluid around the heart. About 7% of patients may develop radiation pneumonitis (inflammation of the lungs) but the patients who develop it usually have a previous lung condition such as asthma. The condition of radiation pneumonitis is also dependent upon the amount of radiation received.[2] Patients with high body mass and previous existing pulmonary or lung disease are most likely to get radiation pneumonitis. This occurs in only occurs in 7% of patients. This is why it is important to make sure that 3-dimensional planning for the radiation treatment is performed to minimize the amount of lung irradiated.

When left sided breast cancers are treated with radiation there may be irradiation to a small amount of the left ventricle or lower chamber of the heart included in the radiation fields. Of the patients who developed radiation pericarditis (inflammation of the sac surrounding the heart and the surface of the heart) 5% or less of the heart's left ventricle was involved and usually over 25 Gy of radiation was received. Approximately 20-50% of patients were found to have vascular (blood vessel) disease.[8] Risk for death due to radiation of the heart during treatment in women who required treatment for left sided breast cancer in the last 30 years has significantly decreased because of three-dimensional radiation treatment and the more focused therapy techniques like balloon Brachytherapy and improvements in cardiovascular (heart blood vessel) treatments.

The most common minor and general side effects of radiation treatment is fatigue. This is may be due to a low red blood cell count, the patient's nutritional status, pain, post chemotherapy status, clinical depression and stress. If the fatigue is caused by a low red blood cell count Procrit can be prescribed to stimulate the body to produce more red blood cells. Make sure your physician or the radiation treatment nurse knows of your symptoms. Nutritional support can easily be added to your treatment as well as a good exercise program to lessen your stress and increase your strength and endurance.

Another side effect of radiation is that of loss of skin integrity. Treatment plans usually call for treatment Monday through Friday for 5 days. The first noticeable changes may be some reddening of the skin, some soreness and darkening and shininess of the skin or atrophy. By four weeks the skin may become dry and scaly. It is important to administer moisturizing lotions or oils with vitamin E to help the skin integrity. On later treatments if the skin may becomes weepy, let your physician know of this condition. The remaining treatments are usually postponed until the skin is healed. Hyperpigmentation of the skin, increase browning or darkening of the skin occurs with minor scaling and dryness may last up to five years post radiation treatment.

References:
1. Jagsi R, Powell S, et al. A Local regional recurrence rates and prognostic factors for failure of node-negative patients treated with mastectomy alone implications for post-mastectomy irradiation. Int J Radiation Oncol Biol Phys. 2003; 57(2 suppl)S128.

2. Allen AM, Prosnitz RG et al. Body mass index predicts the incidence of radiation pneumonitis in node-positive breast cancer. Int J Radiat Oncol Biol Phys. 2003; 57(2 suppl)S130.

3.Fisher B, Dignam J, Wolmark N, Mamounas E, Costantino J, Poller W, et al. Lumpectomy and radiation therapy for the treatment of intraductal breast cancer findings from National Surgical Adjuvant Breast and Bowel Project B-17. J Clin Oncol 1998,16:441-52.

4. Overgaard M, Hansen PS, Overgaard J, Rose C, Andersson M, Bach F, et al. Postoperative radiotherapy in high-risk premenopausal women with breast cancer who receive adjuvant chemotherapy. Danish Breast Cancer Cooperative Group 82b trial. N Engl J Med 1997,337:949-55. 5.

5. Overgaard M, Jensen MB, Overgaard J, Hansen PS, and Rose C, and Andersson M, et al. Postoperative radiotherapy in high-risk postmenopausal breast-cancer patients given adjuvant tamoxifen Danish Breast Cancer Cooperative Group DBCG 82c randomized trial. Lancet 1999,353:1641-8.

6. Thieriault, R. Breast cancer treatment safe during pregnancy, mothers and infants can both do well, new research suggests. Health Day News. June 23, 2006.

7. Vaidya JS, et al "Targeted intraoperative radiotherapy versus whole breast radiotherapy for breast cancer (TARGIT-A trial): an international, prospective, randomsed, non-inferiority phase 3 trial" Lancet 2010; DOI: 10.1016/S0140-6736(10)60837-9.

8. Marks LB, Yu X et al. The impact of irradiated left ventricular volume on the incidence of radiation-induced cardiac perfusion changes. Int J Radiat Oncol Biol phys. *2003, 57(2 suppl)S129.*

Lessons To Be Learned

1) Ask your radiation oncologist (physician) what type of treatments you will receive.
2) Ask your doctor whether or not these treatments will cure you.
3) Ask how many treatments you will receive, how often and how long the treatments will last.
4) Learn how to take care of your skin during and after treatment?
5) Ask your physician how the treatment will affect your skin or other parts of your body and how long these changes will last.

5) Be familiar of what types of side effects the treatment may have.
6) Know whom you should call if you experience a side effect of the treatment.
7) Ask you doctor whether or not you need to come back for a check up after the treatments are over.

SURGICAL RECONSTRUCTION

Many patients treated for breast cancer will elect to have breast conserving surgery (BCS). The cosmetic appearance of this technique is good and the breast is not disfigured by large scars left by mastectomy. Patients undergoing this technique have the same experience with recurrence as patients that undergo mastectomy. It is extremely important for patients treated by this method to receive the same amount of counseling as patients undergoing mastectomy and be advised as to what the breast may look like after their surgery. Minimal asymmetry of the breasts may be acceptable to most patients, but more pronounced asymmetry of the breasts has been associated with depression in some 34% of patients. [1]

Contraindications to breast conservation surgery (BCS) or skin sparing mastectomy :

   -Multiple primary breast tumors in different quadrants of the breast
   -Repeat lumpectomies where the tumor was not completely removed
   - Diffuse mammographic microcalcifications
   - Previous history of radiation to the breast
   - Patient unable to lie flat or grasp and move their arm
   - Tumor in a breast of small size
   - Breast tumors larger than 5 cm (2 inches)
   - Pregnant women
   - Autoimmune or collagen vascular disease (lupus or scleroderma)
   - Obesity with markedly enlarged breasts.

Approximately 17% of patients diagnosed with breast cancer in the United States will elect to have breast reconstruction. Breast reconstruction has become an essential part of the treatment for breast cancer. Its main objective is to improve the quality of woman's life.[2] The diagnosis of breast cancer to a woman may carry with it psychological effects that may be devastating. It is extremely important that as a patient you take time to determine whether or not reconstruction is right for you.

If you decide to have reconstruction your surgeon will help you to determine what reconstructive procedure may be the best for you. All women are different in stature, body fat, muscle mass and breast size and the type of procedure recommended may be based upon these differences. If you determine that reconstruction is best for you, it is important that you let your surgeon, oncologist and radiation oncologist know so that a treatment plan can be best tailored for you.

The past fifty years have brought radical changes in how breast cancer is treated. Rarely is a radical mastectomy performed. Today skin-sparing mastectomies are performed when there is no direct tumor, cancer spread or invasion of the skin. The surgeon usually makes an oblique or horizontal elliptical incision to remove the breast tissue, the nipple or areola and the original biopsy scar. The nipple may also be spared in some cases. Small tumors can be removed by a surgical cut or incision around the areola. Sentinel node biopsies are now routinely performed to preserve the axillary lymphatic system and eliminate the risk of lymphedema (swelling of the arm). The preservation of the skin envelope and the inframammary fold or crease below the breast are essential in breast reconstruction.

The trend in the country currently is for more immediate reconstruction. In a report from MD Anderson Cancer Center in 1990-1993, 54 patients underwent radical mastectomy and 50% had locally advanced disease. Reconstruction did not adversely effect postoperative radiation and chemotherapy treatments. Relapse or recurrence rates were similar to other patients not having reconstruction. [3] The timing of the reconstruction surgery is important. You must discuss the timing with your physicians (surgeon, oncologist and radiation oncologist), so than your treatment plan is tailored to meet your specific treatment needs, based on your tumor size, and stage of disease.

Types of Reconstruction Procedures

Implant reconstruction (submuscular implant)   Breast reconstruction using an implant is chosen in 75% of patients and is the simplest procedure. In the first step of the reconstruction process, a tissue expander or envelope filled with saline is placed beneath the pectoralis chest muscle. It can be filled with additional saline fluid after the procedure. The procedure may be done as an outpatient electively after the completion of chemotherapy or immediately after mastectomy in patients with ductal carcinoma in situ (DCIS) or locally advanced disease. Additional fluid may be added each week and after 3 to 4 weeks the expander is removed and the permanent saline or silicone gel implant inserted. Several months later a nipple is constructed using a strip-flap of skin. It is usually obtained from the highest aspect of medial inner thigh near the labia majora. The skin in this area is more hyperpigmented in all races. Some surgeons may elect to make the nipple and the areola using the same skin and others may prefer to make the areola three months later by tattooing.

Submuscular Implant Figure 23.1

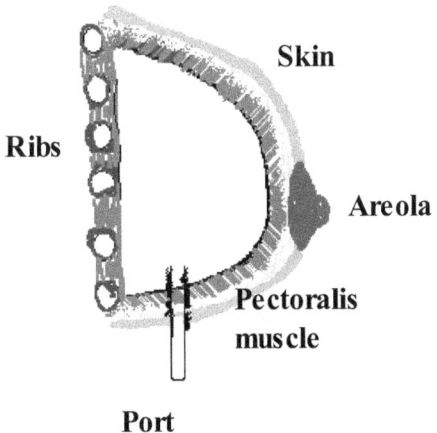

Reconstruction following mastectomy has been found to be safe and beneficial. [4] Cancer relapse or recurrence rates for patients undergoing immediate construction with locally advanced disease and those with delayed reconstruction is similar. Again as stated previously, whether or not to have immediate reconstruction or delayed reconstruction is a decision, which has to be made by you as the patient in consultation with your physicians. For some women a delayed reconstruction may be more appropriate especially where there is extensive tumor involvement of the breast and lymph nodes or when there is inflammatory carcinoma of the breast. It is more likely that such women will undergo extensive postoperative chemotherapy and radiation therapy and will then be assessed for reconstruction post treatment.

Types of Implants

Saline implants are a synthetic product with a short lifespan. Ninety-seven percent of the implants survive 10 years. If the implant ruptures, the normal saline is absorbed into the tissues and is not harmful. Ruptured implants should be removed as soon as possible to lessen the susceptibility to infection. Implants have been removed that had the bacteria, Actinomycetes and fungi growing within the capsule. Women with saline-filled implants that have deflated must have re-operation.

In the past it was thought that **Silicone gel-filled** implants were associated with a significant increased in the risk of the development of the so-called autoimmune disorders or connective diseases like systemic lupus erythematosis (SLE) or Lupus, scleroderma, Sjorgens syndrome, and mixed connective tissue disorders. Literature in the past 10 years has not found a significant increase in these disorders over the general population.

Implants may have a cellular inflammatory reaction at the capsule surface. The body may form a dense fibrous capsule or wall around the implant. Contractures of the capsule of the implant occur in 50% of the silicone gel implants and in 16% of the saline implants. [5] The capsular contractures cause a dense fibrous scar tissue around the implant, tightening and squeezing it. What may be noticed is a soreness and increased firmness in the area of the breast. The breast may look normal and feel soft or may be slightly firm or very firm and look abnormal, or it may be painful, hard and abnormal. [5] Radiologic techniques by mammography, ultrasound and MRI may verify the presence of the capsule rupture, but false negative and false positive results do occur. The most definitive way to diagnose a leak is to surgically remove the implant.

Breast implants do not last forever and most probably will have a complication for which they will eventually have to be removed. There may be a series of physical examinations and reoperations because of the complications particularly if changes are cosmetically undesirable. You need to be aware that the breast implantation may not be a one-time surgery and that implants are not lifetime devices and that you may have to have the implant removed and replaced.

Table 23.1.

Reasons for non-surgical treatments and reoperations and/or removal of breast implants	
Asymmetry	Inflammation or irritation
Breast pain	Malposition/displacement
Breast tissue atrophy	Necrosis
Calcification	Breast and nipple change
Capsular contracture	Palpability/visibility
Chest wall deformity	Ptosis or sagging
Delayed wound healing	Redness or bruising
Extrusion	Rupture/deflation
Galactorrhea	Scarring
Granuloma	Seroma
Hematoma	Patient dissatisfaction
Injury	Wrinkling/dimpling
Infection [5]	

Implants may affect your ability to produce breast milk. You may still get sagging breasts even with the implant. Your health insurance premiums may increase if you have reconstruction or implantation. If there are treatment complications they may not be covered by insurance and you may be dropped or denied health insurance in the future. Implants may not be safe in patients with previous existing autoimmune diseases, like systemic lupus erythematosis (SLE) or lupus and scleroderma, bad wound healing, blood clotting disorders and a weakened immune system. The implants interfere with mammographic examination and make it difficult to examine the breasts. The compression applied to the breasts during mammography may cause the implant to rupture. If you perform Breast self-examinations each month you should also perform it on the breast with the implant checking for any new lumps. Any new lumps or bumps and sores should be evaluated by your physician. [6]

AUTOLOGOUS TISSUE RECONSTRUCTION
(The TRAM, DIEP and GAP Flaps)

Autologous tissue reconstruction is using one's own tissue to reconstruct the breast. The three main autologous reconstruction types are the TRAM, DIEP and GAP flaps. The **latissimus dorsi myocutaneous (TRAM)** flap was the method of choice for breast reconstruction in 1977. This surgical procedure uses the latissimus dorsi muscle of the back with overlying skin this is then transferred from the back to the breast area for reconstruction. A tissue expander implant is placed beneath the flap to provide bulk and 3 months later the expander is replaced with a permanent saline or silicone implant. The flap procedure can be done immediately after mastectomy or delayed. The downside of this procedure is that the scar will be visible in low cut dresses and swimwear. There is loss of function of a large muscle from the back and if there is a complication with the implant a reoperation will be required. One-third of the implants that are removed are from patients with latissimus flaps.

The **transverse rectus abdominis musculocutaneous (TRAM)** flap in 1982 was the method of choice for autologous tissue breast reconstruction in the United States. It consists of a skin ellipse and the underlying subcutaneous tissue beneath the skin from the mid-abdomen attached to pedicle of rectus abdominus muscle with the superior epigastric artery and the internal mammary arteries as principal blood supply. The flap is tunneled from the abdomen to the chest to make a new breast. It is superior to the latissimus dorsi myocutaneous flap since it can provide a satisfactory cosmetic effect with a permanent lifetime result without the use of implants. The downside of the procedure is that it uses the abdominal muscles and may lead to weakness of the muscles of the abdomen and result in hernias. The complication rate is about 20%.

The **deep inferior epigastric perforator procedure (DIEP)** is a refinement of the TRAM. It consists of skin and the subcutaneous fatty tissue and takes no abdominal muscle. It does not rely on microsurgery to move tiny blood vessels. This procedure is preferable than the TRAM in that patients experience less abdominal wall weakness, pain and functional difficulties. The abdominal contour or shape is usually improved. [7] Despite this the TRAM flap procedure remains the procedure of choice for patients who want autologous tissue reconstruction because it provides the most satisfactory breast form with a permanent result. [8]

TRAM

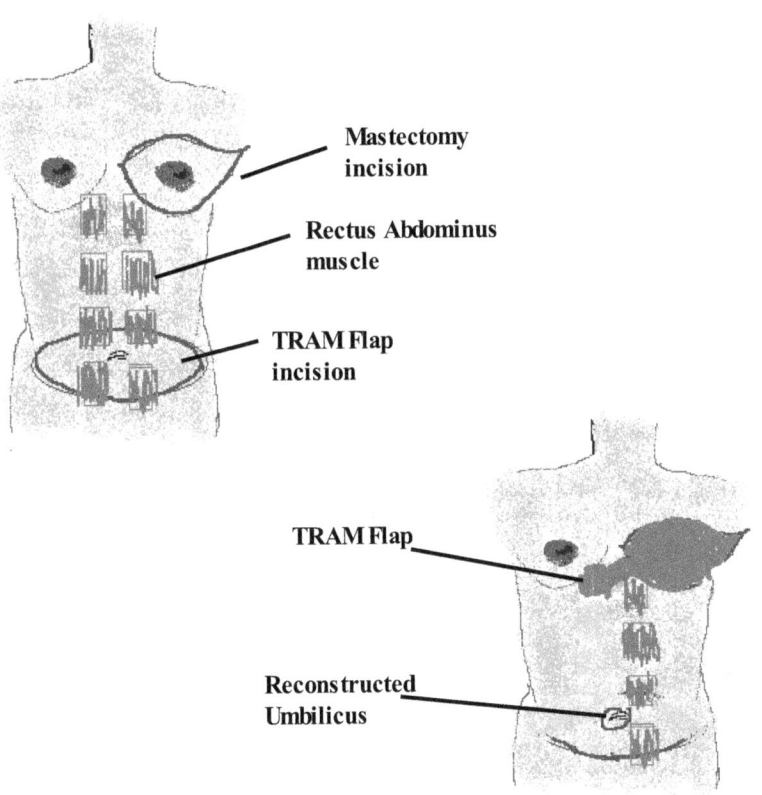

Mastectomy
incision

Rectus Abdominus
muscle

TRAM Flap
incision

TRAM Flap

Reconstructed
Umbilicus

Figure 23.2.

For about 20% of patients undergoing mastectomy, the abdomen is not a suitable donor site. The **superior gluteal artery perforator flap (S-GAP)** was introduced by Fujino uses buttocks fat which may be a suitable alternative site for autologous tissue for reconstruction. The S-GAP procedure meets patient satisfaction but is difficult to perform   and vein grafts are needed. It is used as an alternative site for postmastectomy reconstruction in tall thin or athletic women of average body mass and in patients who have failed a previous reconstruction with implants or have inadequate abdominal tissue for reconstruction. [9]

DIEP

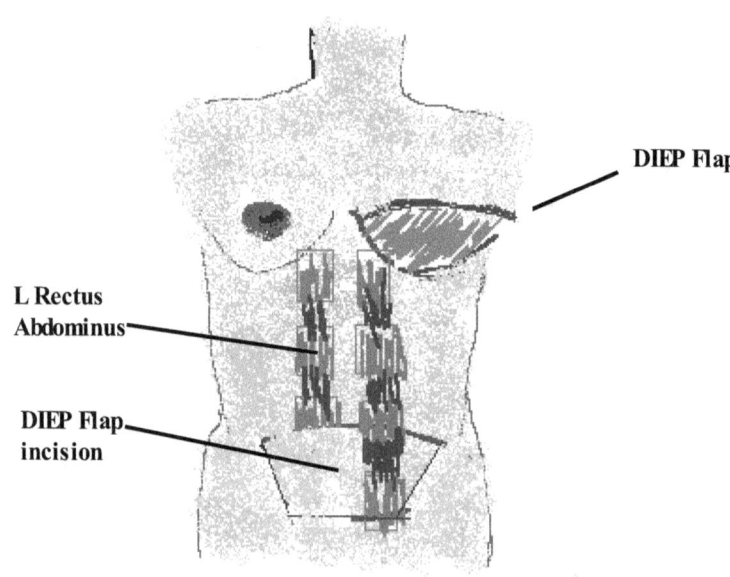

Figure 23.3

Both the DIEP and S-GAP flaps have a 99% success rate. The DIEP and S-GAP procedures are three stage procedures. The first stage is performed immediately after mastectomy and restores breast volume and shape allowing the patient to fit into a normal bra. The second stage is 8 weeks after the first and may be delayed until chemotherapy or radiation is completed. This is the stage of nipple reconstruction. The third stage is 8 weeks after the second stage and consists of medical tattooing of the areola or skin around the nipple to restore pigment.

Breast reconstruction rarely produces a result that is completely symmetrical to the other unaffected breast. The implants that are used in the procedure are for a B or C cup and reconstruction cannot produce a pendulous breast. The unaffected breast may have to undergo mammoplasty (breast reduction) and a breast lift procedure may have to be performed on the large pendulous breast in order to produce the best cosmetic effect. Small breasts cannot be reconstructed by the TRAM procedure, because the reconstructed breast would be larger than the other unaffected breast and augmentation (plastic surgery enhancement) of unaffected breast would be necessary. Submuscular implants also make mammographic examination of the breast difficult especially when a capsule develops around the implant.

Summary

Most women who undergo mastectomy also have breast reconstruction. The most common procedure is reconstruction by submuscular implants and autologous tissue reconstruction. The TRAM reconstruction procedure is preferred by plastic surgeons because the DIEP and S-GAP are procedures are complex and microsurgery techniques are required. Techniques used for reconstruction are based on the patient's medical condition, stage of disease, body habitus and the need for postoperative chemotherapy or neoadjuvant chemotherapy and radiation.

Breast sparing surgeries have completely transformed the treatment of breast cancer and have been proven to be a safe alternative to mastectomy, but mastectomy may still be indicated in patients with multiple tumors or large tumors in the breast, and in multicentric ductal carcinoma in situ, DCIS. Breast reconstruction should be considered and discussed prior to the first surgical procedure so that the you may have a realistic perception of what are the advantages of breast reconstruction and what procedures may be involved in the reconstruction process. Reconstruction is based on individual body habitus, stage of disease and whether or not the procedure may be more advantageous to be immediately performed or delayed because of additional therapies or other health conditions. Outcomes have shown that immediate reconstruction is safe and that it does have the advantage of early return to ones lifestyle, personal freedom and self image. The outcome is immediate rather than deferred. Most women prefer the immediate procedure rather than the delayed procedure for this reason.

References:

1. Waljee JF, et al "The effect of aesthetic outcome following breast conserving surgery on psychosocial functioning and quality of life" *J Clin Oncol* 2008; 26: epub.
2. Mammoplasty-mastectomy. Gynecol Obstret Fertility. 2003.June, 31(5):574. Montpellier, France.
3. Newman LA, Luerer HM et al. Feasibility of immediate breast reconstruction for locally advanced breast cancer. Ann Surg Oncol. 1999, 6:671-675.
4. Alan R. Shons, MD, PhD, Marseille g, et al. Postmastectomy breast reconstruction Current techniques. Cancer Control 8(5)419-426. 2001. H. Lee Moffitt Cancer Center and Research Institute, Inc. Abstract
5. Plast Reconstr Surg 1990; 86809-11.
6. Berwick, Carly. Ideas and Resources for recovery reconstruction refined/ MAMM; vol (2); No12, 1999.
7. Gylbert L, Asplund O, Jurell G. Capsular formation after breast reconstruction with silicone-gel and saline-filled implants a 6-year follow-up
8. Guerra, AB, Metzinger SE, et al. Breast reconstruction with Gluteal Artery perforator Flaps. Annals of Plastic Surgery,52:(2)p.118-125. Feb 2004.
9. Safety of Silicone Breast Implants. Institute of Medicine National Academy Press, Washington, DC(IOM Report).
10. Futter CM, Webster MH, Hagen S, et al. A retrospective comparison of abdominal muscle strength following breast reconstruction with a free TRAM or DIEP flap. Br J Plast Surg. 2000,53:578-583.

11. Mentor and McGhan's patient's brochure.
(http://www.fda.gov/cdrh/whatsnew)

Lessons To Be Learned
1) If your surgeon suggests mastectomy as part of your treatment plan ask him the reason for this decision and whether or not there are any other options. Ask for a second opinion if you are not convinced that you need a mastectomy.
2) If you are considering breast reconstruction ask for a consultation to see a surgeon who specializes in breast reconstruction.
3) Ask about the types of reconstruction and go over what type of reconstruction that the surgeon feels may be best for you and be sure to ask why.
4) Be informed of the complications that may occur because of the procedure.
5) Ask to see pictures of patients and examples of reconstruction surgeries that the surgeon has performed.
6) Ask the surgeon if he has any patients that would not mind speaking to you about how they felt about their surgery.

PALLIATIVE THERAPY

Palliative therapy is the care or treatment given to cancer patients to reduce the severity of disease symptoms, pain and suffering in order to improve the quality of life of those facing life threatening diseases. This care may occur during or after treatment of the disease and while the patient struggles to survive the impact of the disease and its treatment. It also includes the care given after surviving treatment, the care if and when the disease recurs, the suffering which occurs during the advanced stage of disease and end of life care or hospice care. The following will be discuss: treatment of the side effects of chemotherapy, radiation therapy, adjuvant hormonal therapy menopausal symptoms, pain control, physical therapy, anxiety and depression, counseling, and hospice care.

Chemotherapy Side Effects

Fever

Hyperthermia or fever is commonly found in patients with cancer. The following may be causes of elevated temperature: infections, paraneoplastic syndrome (symptoms associated with the tumor), neuroleptic malignant syndrome (hyperthermia or high fever due to anesthesia) and blood product usage. Symptoms can include tiredness, muscle aches and pains, sweating and chills. Infections may occur in cancer patients because of leukopenia or low white blood cell count caused by the destruction of white blood cells from chemotherapy. Symptoms related to an infection may be that of fever, sweating, chills, tiredness, muscle aches and pains, diarrhea, shortness of breath, skin rashes or redness of the skin, low blood pressure, an abscess of the skin or an infection which is more deep in the skin or one the body cavities or mouth or oral cavity.

If the white blood cell count is low the oncologist may prescribe Neupogen to increase the white cell count and ward off infection. If an infection has occurred it may be usually caused by gram-negative or gram-positive staining bacteria, but predominantly by gram positive Staphylococci or Streptococci. The source of infection may be due to an infected vascular device or catheter, or possibly the Port-a-cath, which may need to be removed. Prophylactic antibiotics can be given. Occasionally infections are due to gram-negative bacteria and such infections may be more difficult to treat if the organisms are resistant to multiple antibiotics.

Stomatitis is infections and sores of the surfaces of the mouth, or cheeks, gums lips, tongue and throat. If you have sores in your mouth, feel pain when you eat, have a dry mouth or notice changes in taste and smell you should bring it to the attention of your oncology doctor or nurse. Stomatitis can be treated with mouth rinses. For preventive measure good oral hygiene is necessary. Brush your teeth and tongue after each meal and before sleep using tooth paste with fluoride and baking soda. Use mouth washes containing ¼ teaspoon baking soda and 1/8 teaspoon of salt in a cup of warm water several times a day. Keep your mouth moist. Do not use tobacco or other products. Do not drink alcohol. Do not eat any foods that may injure your mouth, like popcorn or chips or crunchy foods. Limit sugary foods and acidic foods. If you develop a significant infection of the mouth your doctor may prescribe a mucositis/stomatitis combination oral medication for the infection. Use a lip balm to prevent chapped lips. Similarly the esophagus may develop a mucositis as well as the intestines. This may feel as though the insides of your chest and belly are hot. Your physician can prescribe mixture of Maalox, lidocaine (a pain medication) and Benadryl (an antihistamine). If you have an infection caused by the yeast Candida, the drug Nystatin may be prescribed.

Fever can also be caused by bowel, bladder and kidney obstructions or blockages due to spread of the tumor. Bleeding into the brain and other organs and clotting of blood vessels, autoimmune or connective tissue disorders can also cause fever. Your doctor will discover the source of the fever in order to appropriately treat the you. Your physician will perform a thorough physical exam, collect urine and blood cultures and examine catheters and tubes that may be attached you to find the cause. After the underlying cause is treated, fluids are usually given in the vein for hydration (the body's water balance), as well as food for nutritional support and other palliative treatment as needed. Clinical syndromes associated with cancer that may cause fever can easily be treated with nonsteroidal anti-inflammatory drugs like Tylenol, Advil, or Ibuprofen.

Certain drugs, narcotics and benzodiazepines(Valium, Librum, etc.) may cause neuroleptic malignant syndrome which is associated with high fever, nausea and vomiting, delirium, muscle rigidity, instability and confusion can be treated by supportive therapy and discontinuation of the offending drugs. Fevers associated with the use of blood products or transfusions can be decreased if white blood cell poor blood products are given. These fevers are usually treated with Benadryl or Tylenol. [1,2]

Nausea and Vomiting

Nausea and vomiting induced by chemotherapy is an accepted effect of treatment for breast cancer, but there are things that can be done to lessen these side effects and anxieties that you may experience to improve your quality of life. The nausea and vomiting experienced during the first day of chemotherapy is probably anticipatory. If everyone tells you that you are going to have nausea and vomiting and that this is what you should expect, you will have nausea and vomiting on the first round of treatments and in successive rounds unless it is controlled on the first round of treatment.

The chemotherapy drugs Adriamycin and Cyclophosphamide are used to treat breast cancer patients. The levels of these drugs are much increase on the first day of treatment and decrease on the following days post treatment so the rational should be that nausea and vomiting should decrease on successive days, but that is not the case. Many patients have nausea and vomiting while the levels of the drug and decreasing. Most experience it 2-3 days after infusion of the chemotherapy drugs. Nausea and vomiting tends to be experienced more in women than men. Younger women are more likely to experience these side effects than older women and women who have experienced these symptoms during pregnancy are more likely to experience these symptoms than women who have not been pregnant.

Your doctor will select a drug that will be most protective for the treatment of any nausea or vomiting that you may experience. There are several classes of drugs used. Compazine and serotonin-receptor antagonist drugs are the most common anti-nausea and anti-emetic (anti-vomiting) drugs used to treat nausea and vomiting. The most common serotonin-receptor antagonists used are Dolastrin, Granisetron,

Ondansetron and Palonosetron. Theses drugs have not been found to help delayed nausea and vomiting significantly. The drug Aprepitant is in a new drug class, the neurokinin-1 (NK-1 receptor antagonists). It is usually prescribed along with steroids and a serotonin antagonist and helps in relieving the delayed symptoms of nausea. Emend is a newer drug that helps prevents first day nausea and vomiting up to five days after the administration of the chemotherapy drugs. Fosapritant has also been found to be effective. As newer agents are developed, the guidelines for treatment will change. More research must be done to control delayed nausea and identify the trigger factors that induce the symptoms.

Drugs with antiemetic activity   Table 24.1

Drug class	Drug
Phenothiazines	Chlorpromazine Prochlorperazine
Substituted benzamide	Metoclopramide
Antihistamines	Benadryl
Corticosteroid	Dexamethasone
Anticholinergic	Scopolamine
Cannabinoid	Nabilone
5-HT$_3$ (serotonin) receptor antagonist	Granisetron
Benzodiazepine	Lorazepam
NK$_1$receptor antagonist	Aprepitant

Marijuana has been used in supportive care for some cancer patients to alleviate nausea and vomiting and anorexia, loss of appetite. Prescription for the use of marijuana or the pill form delta-9-tetrahydrocannabinol (THC) as an anti-emetic are available for those patients who have not responded to standard therapy. [3]   The use of marijuana must be weighed against its side effects. More studies must be done to fully evaluate whether or not it is effective in the supportive care of patients and whether or not it is of value in improving the quality of life in patients who have anorexia and cachexia (muscle wasting) with extreme weight loss. [4]

If you do not experience significant nausea and vomiting, but experience occasional symptoms, you can lie down and put a cool cloth on your forehead to keep you from thinking about being nauseous. Avoid noxious or unpleasant odors, tobacco smoke, perfumes, cleaning supplies or chemicals that may make you want to vomit. The chemotherapy drug Cytoxan makes your sense of smell keen and may cause some scents of things in your environment or surrounding to stand out, like plastics which you have never smelled before. Things that you used to liked to smell before like the aroma of coffee may now be a trigger for your nausea. Try to avoid your triggers. Natural remedies that can relieve the urge to vomit such as ginger as a tea or in capsule form and peppermint oil or tea can stop intestinal cramps. There is also some evidence that flavonoid-rich fruit and vegetables i.e. grape juice, oranges, tangerines, grapefruits and other citrus fruits, legumes, grains and nuts may provide some protection against chemotherapy induced nausea and vomiting. If you do vomit, make sure to drink enough water or beverages to replace the amount of fluid that you loss. Chicken and beef broth may ease your stomach as well as clear beverages like Seven-up, ginger ale, teas and water. Pasta, noodles, oatmeal, cream of wheat, crackers and pretzels, plain white rice, potatoes, and baked chicken may be more palatable. Bananas, canned fruits and jello may also be soothing. If your symptoms are severe and your bouts of vomiting are frequent and you cannot eat, or if your daily routine has been interrupted or if you become weak and dizzy contact your doctor immediately.

Alopecia (Hair Loss)

The hair loss from chemotherapy is temporary. The chemotherapy drugs Adriamycin and Taxol cause complete hair loss and Cytoxan causes minimal hair loss. As we have stated before, chemotherapy affects both cancer cells and normal cells in the S and M phases of the cell cycle.

Chemotherapy destroys cancer cells and normal cells alike and is indiscriminant. The hair follicles of the skin have cells that rapidly grow and reproduce every 23 to 72 hrs. These rapidly producing normal cells are destroyed just like the cancer cells. Within 2 weeks after the start of chemotherapy all body hair is loss. Hair loss can be quite disfiguring and depressing for most women. You can hide the loss of a breast with your clothing, but hair loss is apparent to everyone who sees you. Some women elect to go out in public bald, but a lot of women cannot do this. Some women can do creative things with the head scarves and turbans that may cause others to not notice the hair loss. They may consider the turban or scarf to be part of a chic way of dressing. There are turbans and hats available the have a fringe of hair along the top or sides, but you should look for at the quality of the fringe of hair before you considering buying them. There are also some caps with pony tails attached to them that are good if you are just going on a short run or to your child's baseball or soccer game.

Good quality wigs are available. Before the start of chemotherapy consider contacting you stylist or a wig specialist. You may be able to choose a wig and have it styled to look exactly like your hair, so that when you do lose your hair no one will notice. You can by real hair, but these wigs are expensive. There are excellent quality synthetic wigs available. The best synthetic wigs are : Raquel Welch, Noriko, Renee of Paris, Amore Designer, and Revlon. Beverly Johnson, Sepia and Motown Tress make wigs for African Americans. These wigs can be ordered by your wig stylist or online through the internet. It is best however, to have a stylist style the wig once you receive.

You can also consider having your hair cut short before therapy begins and then going to a short style wig that is similar to your short hairdo or consider having you head shaven immediately so that you do not have to go through the trauma of seeing your hair fall out and have a wig styled for you immediately. If you decide on a short hairdo, it will be easy for you to wear your own hair when it begins to grow back.

Table 24.2 *229*

TREATMENT OF SIDE EFFECTS OF CHEMOTHERAPY

SYMPTOMS	TREATMENT
Alopecia	Cessation of chemotherapy
Allergic reactions	Corticosteroids, Benadryl
Anemia	Procrit
Leukopenia	Neupogen
Arthralgia (joint pain)	Tylenol or Advil, NSAIDs
Diarrhea	Treatment of infection with antibiotics and fluid replacement
Nausea and vomiting	Antiemetics, Benadryl, Lorazepam
Shortness of breath	Exam for lung and heart disease, pulmonary disease, pneumonia, embolism, cardiotoxicity, MI
Weakness	Access diet and rest
Peripheral nerve damage	Glutamine with oxidizers
Skin rashes	Antibiotics, Antifungal or steroid cremes, supportive care
Erythema of skin	Rule out infection, antibiotics, supportive care, steroids
Liver dysfunction	Evaluation of liver disease
Hypotension	Treatment of causes cardiovascular, infection and fluid loss
Abscess	Incision and drainage and antibiotics
Phlebitis	Antibiotics, antitoxin
Stomatitis (mouth infection)	Mouth rinses

230 **Abdominal cramps**	**Rule out food poisoning or infection, antibiotics**
Irregular menstrual periods	**Cessation of chemotherapy, check platelet count**
Nail discoloration and thickening	**Cessation of chemotherapy**
Fatigue	**Rest and/or treatment of anemia**
Esophagitis	**Anti-acids and or antifungals**
Discolored urine	**Rule out blood in urine**
Painful urination	**Antibiotics for infection**
Hyperuricemia (gout)	**Colchicine**
Stomach ulcers	**Anti-acids**
Pericarditis	**Antibiotics, corticosteroids**
Thrombocytopenia	**Platelets**

Radiation Side Effects

The most common minor side effects of radiation treatment is fatigue, this is also the most common general side effect of radiation treatment. This is may be due to a low red blood cell count, the patient's nutritional status, pain, post chemotherapy status, clinical depression and stress. If the fatigue is caused by a low red blood cell count the drug, Procrit can be prescribed to stimulate the body to produce more red blood cells. Make sure your physician or the radiation treatment nurse knows of your symptoms. Nutritional support can easily be added to your treatment as well as a good exercise program to lessen your fatigue and increase your strength and endurance.

Another side effect of radiation is that of the loss of skin integrity. Treatment plans usually call for treatment Monday through Friday for 5 days. The first noticeable skin changes that may occur are some reddening of the skin, possible soreness, darkening and shininess of the skin or atrophy. By four weeks the skin may become dry and scaly. It is important to administer moisturizing lotions or oils with vitamin E to help the skin integrity. On later treatments if the skin may becomes weepy, let your physician knows of this condition. Treatments are usually discontinued until the skin is healed. Hyperpigmentation of the skin, the increased browning or darkening of the skin occurs with minor scaling and dryness for several years after radiation treatment.

Adjuvant Hormonal Therapy Menopausal Symptoms

Women who have histories of hormone replacement therapy are at an increased risk for breast cancer, coronary heart disease, blood clots strokes, senile dementia or Alzheimer's disease. Women who have had breast cancer and are at increased risk for breast cancer recurrence. Breast cancer is a contraindication to hormonal therapy and alternatives to hormone therapy are advised for women with breast cancer. The breast cancer patient who has had either invasive ductal carcinoma or invasive lobular carcinoma or tubular and who may be either premenopausal or on hormonal therapy for menopausal symptoms is at higher risk for the recurrence than the postmenopausal women. Medium potency estrogen-progestin therapy has been more strongly associated with lobular carcinoma. Tubular carcinoma is associated with medium potency estrogen-progestin therapy and alcohol.[5] It is not known whether or not estrogen alone causes this increase or if it is just the medium potency estrogen-progestin combination. Further research is being conducted to determine this.

Current breast cancer treatment is base upon the ER and PR status of the tumor. The use of anti-estrogens like tamoxifen and newer drugs exacerbate the symptoms of hot flashes and night sweats, vaginal dryness, sleep disturbance, and osteoporosis. The standard treatment for the non-breast cancer patient for hot flashes has been the use of estrogen by itself or with progestin as an effective way to reduce the symptoms, but this cannot be used in women who have had breast cancer. There must be alternatives.

It is believed that hot flashes are triggered by elevations in the body core temperature which causes blood vessels to dilate or the opening of the vessel to widen when a set upper temperature is reached and decrease when a set lower temperature is reached. If the temperature zone is narrowed, then when a small elevation of the body core temperature occurs, and hot flashes are triggered. [8] A hot flash may last as long as a few seconds to up to six minutes.

Symptoms can range from hot flashes without sweating, hot flashes with sweating not limiting activity, and hot flashes with profuse sweating that may cause a woman to stop activities. The sweating can be so severe at night that sleep problems occur and insomnia develops. If you go to bed at 10:00 PM and awake at 3:00 AM and your night clothes are soaking wet and you can't get back to sleep you may be experiencing severe symptoms. If you have a hot flash while driving a car in the winter time and turn on the air conditioner freezing out your spouse and the other passengers in the car who decide to put on their winter coats, or if your are at work and suddenly can't concentrate on the task at hand because of hot flashes then maybe you are experiencing severe symptoms.

Studies have been conducted to determine whether or not there were any factors of living that could be modified to reduce hot flashes. It was found that factors were different for premenopausal and postmenopausal patients. A high dietary fat intake in the postmenopausal woman correlated with hot flashes. So decreasing the amount of fat in the diet could decrease the amount of hot flashes. In the premenopausal woman a high body mass resulted in increased hot flashes and an increased body core temperature because of insulating body fat. Cigarette smoking also increases the risk of hot flashes possibly because of the thermogenic or warming effects of nicotine. In both premenopausal and postmenopausal women the factors of age, race, contraceptive and hormonal replacement use, and depression are not factors that can be modified to reduce hot flashes. [6]

How do you treat hot flashes without using estrogen and progestin? You can reduce the temperature threshold by reducing the temperature of your environment, but if you have others living with you that might not be an acceptable alternative. You can use fans and turn on the air conditioner to low. I must warn you though that keeping temperatures frigid in your bedroom may move your spouse to the next room. You can try eating ice chips. I now know why my mother ate a lot of ice. Ice and cold drinks tend to lower body core temperature. You can also try dressing in layers and reduce the amount of clothing that you have on when needed. If you are a smoker, quit smoking. If you have increased insulation or body fat, go on a weight reduction program. Weight loss in overweight women results on improvement in flushing control.

The withdrawal and lack of estrogen is not the only cause of hot flashes. Researchers have found that levels of methoxy-4-hydroxyphenylglycol (MHPG) which is a brain metabolite or breakdown product of norepinephrine (NE), a brain neurotransmitter or compound that aids in conducting nerve impulses, are elevated before and after the hot flashes in symptomatic women. Clonidine, a drug that reduces the brain NE significantly reduces NE in symptomatic women.[7] Clonidine is effective treatment for hot flashes in breast cancer patients. Clonidine increases the temperature threshold is effective when treating hot flashes when compared to placebos by 89%. It may be taken orally or by transdermal (skin) patches. The side effects of Clonidine include hypotension, dry mouth, rash nausea, gastrointestinal disturbances, some difficulty in sleeping and sedation. When Clonidine was given to patients treated with Tamoxifen the results were conflicting.

The drug Gabapentin has been shown to diminish hot flashes frequency.[9] Gabapentin, an anticonvulsant has also been found to reduce hot flashes by 45%. The mechanism of how it reduces the hot flashes is unknown. The anti-depressant drugs Paroxetine and Venlafaxine also decrease hot flashes. Effexor, Paroxetine, Fluoxetine, Venlafaxine and Citalopram are drugs in the group of selective serotonin (5HT) reuptake inhibitors (SSRIs) drugs which are antidepressants. They have been shown to be effective in treating hot flashes by 40 to 60% when compared to placebos. The side effects are nausea, dry mouth, feeling sleepy, and loss of appetite and insomnia. The newest drug, Citalopram has minimal adverse effects and reduces hot flashes by 46%. It can be given in a low once a day dose and may be taken with Tamoxifen.[10]

Many women report sleep disturbance at menopause. Studies by The Wisconsin Sleep Cohort Study on objective and subjective sleep quality in perimenopausal and postmenopausal women neither provided evidence that hot flashes produce sleep disturbance in symptomatic women nor whether or not treatment of the hot flashes improved sleep.[9] However, now new research has found moderate evidence that menopause can cause sleep disturbances in some women. Sleep disturbance occurs in as much as 42% of perimenopausal women and up to 60% postmenopausal women. Many women report that after surgical menopause, there is a disturbance in their sleep patterns and awakenings and that it is caused by the hot flashes. Researcher M. Ohayon has found that moderate and severe hot flashes were associated with chronic insomnia occurring around or after menopause and states that treating hot flashes could improve sleep quality and minimize chronic insomnia. [14] Estrogen has been found to be helpful for sleep disturbances and mood changes. There be another brain neurotransmitter substance that is produced which impedes the ability of symptomatic women to easily return to sleep after awakenings.

Current literature and the numerous internet websites tend to promote phytoestrogens. There has appeared to be an explosion in the herbal, nutritional and supplemental products marketed to premenopausal and postmenopausal women that are promoted as a means of reducing breast cancer risk and reducing menopausal symptoms. The rational for using phytoestrogens is from the observational comparisons of different societies, i.e. Japanese or Asian diets compared to Western civilization diets, menopausal symptoms and cancer incidence and the assumption that phytoestrogens is the reason for the decreased breast cancer rate and postmenopausal symptoms in Japanese and Asian women. These products are marketed as powders containing isoflavones (Genistein and Daidzein), soy protein, high lignan flaxseed oil, flaxseed, wild yam and roasted soy nuts.

Studies in the mid-1990s have shown a 45% reduction in the number of moderate and severe hot flashes and maturation of the vaginal mucosa in postmenopausal women using these products and this looked promising as a potential to reduce breast cancer risk and bone osteoporosis. [15]   Studies conducted by Stearns et al however, found no improvement in hot flashes relative to placebos. [13] Additional long term studies are needed to determine whether or not these treatments can be recommended as an alternative treatment to traditional hormone replacement therapy and whether or not they have the potential to reduce breast cancer risk. There has been much said on the benefits of soy products and phytoestrogens, red clover leaf, black cohosh, dong quai root, Femtone, Meno-fem, Phyto-est, Phyto-soy, Remifemin in treating hot flashes. However, red clover leaf in studies has not been found to be effective in reducing hot flashes. Don quai root is not effective in the treatment of hot flashes. There is no literature support that Black cohosh is effective in the treatment of hot flashes. Good natural sources of phytoestrogens like alfalfa, apples, green tea, sesame, and wheat which may have some effect on alleviating hot flashes in some women.

Beware of bioidentical hormone products and natural hormone products that are commercially available like Bi-est and Tri-est which contain horse estrogens.[16] Beware of topical estrogens in cosmetics or DHEA creams, progestin and estrogen creams. These bioidentical creams are touted as natural hormones that protect against heart disease, endometrial cancer and breast cancer. Such claims are false. These bioidentical hormones are identical to hormones used by pharmaceutical companies and carry the same risks of heart disease, endometrial cancer and breast cancer. If you have breast cancer stay away from bioidenticals.

PAIN CONTROL

Patients being treated for cancer have the right to have their pain alleviated and to receive medication for their pain. Pain is experienced by at least 30% of cancer patients undergoing treatment for metastatic disease and up to 70% of patients with extensive or advanced disease. [16] Patients and concerned advocates of a friend or loved one need to be informed that the patient has a right to receive medication to alleviate pain, that it is part of the treatment for the pain of cancer, surgery, chemotherapy, radiation treatment, and metastatic or extensive disease. Medications exist to alleviate pain and should be prescribed by your physician without fear of addiction, tolerance or side effects of the medication. Money should not be a factor in whether or not you receive treatment for your pain. The control of pain should receive as much priority as the treatment of the malignancy itself since it can affect the quality of one's life.

The cancer patient does not have to suffer and be in pain. The treatment and the alleviation of pain is part of the treatment plan. If you are having pain let your physician know. Your physician can anticipate conditions in which you may have pain and start you on medication to prevent the pain from starting. If the pain has started and is getting worse your physician can prescribe medications to control the pain. There are many kinds of pain medications, some which may work for you and others that may not.

If you may have had an allergic reaction to a pain medication in the past, it is imperative that you let your physician know. Do not leave out information in your past medical history.

It is extremely important for you and your family to get to know the physicians and nurses those take care of you, so that the right treatment plan can be devised for you. You should feel comfortable enough to speak with your caregivers about your condition. If you experience pain, tell your healthcare provider what type of pain you may be having, whether or not it is constant or intermittent, whether or not it starts at one point in the body and shoots to another part of the body or stays in the same place. You should be able to tell your healthcare provider how often the pain occurs and what you are doing when the pain occurs. You should also tell him whether or not it affects your daily routine and what you can do to make the pain feel better.

Medications Commonly Used for Pain Control

The following medications are used for pain control:
- Mild to moderate pain - Nonsteroidal anti-inflammatory drugs (NSAID) and other non-opioid drugs
- Moderate to severe pain - NSAID plus an opioid
- Severe or unrelieved pain - Highly potent opioids

NSAIDs (nonsteroidal antiflammatory drugs): Aspirin, Celecoxib, Diclofenac, Diflunisal, Fenoprofen, Flurbiprofen, Ibuprofen, Indomethacin, Fenoprofen, and Naproxen

NSAIDs are used in the treatment of mild to moderate pain. NSAIDs can be used to delay the use of opioids and may be effective treatment in organ and bone metastases. NSAIDs are not addictive. The use of NSAIDs with weak opioids for moderate pain is adequate treatment in 60% of patients and for 83% of patients with slightly less than moderate pain. There may be side effects with long-term use of the drugs and risks may exist with usage in the elderly, in patients with kidney and gastrointestinal disease, and when used with other drugs. If you have stomach complaints, let your physician know. There are drugs that your physician can prescribe to prevent gastric and duodenal ulcers that may occur. Anti-acids and over the counter medications do not work, so let your physician know.

OPIOIDS

Morphine is the most frequently used opioid drug for cancer patients with severe or unalleviated pain. Long-term opioid use and the development of tolerance is not linked. The amount of the drug that is needed to alleviate the pain depends on the amount of disease and the individual patient response to the dosage. This is why it is important for you to discuss the amount of pain that you have with your physician and caregivers, because the response to the drugs are variable in each patient. One patient may not respond well to one opioid analgesic but may respond well to a different opioid analgesic. One patient may respond well to the administration of the drug orally by not intravenously. Your physician may have to use an alternate opioid or rotate drugs when one is not effective.

Long Acting Opioids:
SR Morphine, MS Contin, Oramorph SR, and Kadian
SROxycodone, Oxycontin, and newer drugs
Transdermal Fentanyl, Duragesic, SR Hydromorphone, SR Oxymorphone
Methadone, Dolophine

The opioids drugs may be short-acting or long-acting medications. Oxycodone, Methadone and Duragesic are long-acting narcotics. They can control constant pain. The patient with constant pain may have episodes of increased pain, which can be alleviated, with the addition of short-acting medications when necessary. This ensures that the patient is adequately treated and does not get into trouble with substance abuse. Patients who cannot take enough narcotics to alleviate their pain can have a spinal infusion device, which delivers medicine to the space surrounding the spinal cord. Baclofen is usually given. [17] This delivery of the narcotics eliminates the side effects of narcotics.

In extremely difficult cases, Ketamine an anesthetic drug has been found to be effective. A few patients may need spinal treatment, which consists of spinal administration of drugs. Morphine, Bupivacaine and Clonidine have been found to be effective. Nerve blocks and nerve injection treatments may be of some value in some cases. The administrations of Biphosphonates has been found to relieve the pain of bone metastases as well as prevent the development of bone metastases. Invasive breast cancer risk has decreased 33% in postmenopausal women who use biphosphonate drugs.

Massage therapy has been shown to alleviate the pain of arm lymphedema. Cutaneous heat and cold stimulation, exercise, immobilization and transcutaneous nerve stimulation (TENS) and acupuncture have been used and may help in reducing the amount of pain medication needed.

Brain Activation Control

Psychological therapies can be used with analgesics to manage pain. When such treatment is used it does not necessarily mean that the pain was just in the patients mind or not real. Such therapy is being used as a method to help the patient be able to better cope with pain or to develop methods to modify reactions to pain. [19]

Patients with severe pain can learn to control brain activity. Researchers have used real-time functional magnetic resonance imaging to impact or control brain regions involved in pain perception. [20] Patients trained to use automatic feedback mechanisms to control their pain were able to reduce their pain by 64%.

Physical Therapy

Exercise after is imperative no matter what type of surgery you have and especially after breast surgery it affects your arm. It affects the way you move your arm, how you take a deep breath, all of your movements, your day to day activities, personal care and chores. Your doctor can suggest a physical therapist or an occupational therapist that can help you design a special exercise program for you if you do not have full use of your arm 3 weeks after surgery.

Exercise can begin as soon as all drains and sutures are removed. Exercises should be directed to improve arm and shoulder strength and to increase your range of motion. Exercise is a great benefit to the breast cancer patient. Breast cancer patients who exercise 3 to 5 hours a week can cut their risk of dying from breast cancer by 50% when compared to women with sedentary lifestyles. Sedentary lifestyles lead to obesity this leads to higher insulin and insulin-like growth factors that promote the growth of breast cancer. Physical activity decreases the incidence of breast cancer. Moderate aerobic exercise decreases insulin levels and insulin-like growth factors and the risk of recurrence of breast cancer, resulting in a better prognosis for the breast cancer patient.

Anxiety

Just the thought of breast cancer creates anxiety in patients who have their yearly mammogram. How anxious would you be if on touching your breasts you noted a nodule or mass? Would you call your physician immediately or would you deny that the mass is there and neglect your health care and risk your life? Would you fool yourself into believing that the mass is not there and that it has always been there and is normal for your breasts? Would you let your spouse tell you that it is normal even when you know that it isn't let your spouse be co-dependent in your denial and reasoning that if I say it isn't there, and if my spouse says that it isn't there, then it isn't there and it is just my runaway imagination that it is their in the first place.

How anxious are you when you go to your physician for the results of your regularly scheduled mammogram? Imagine your anxiety being compounded when your physician tells you that the radiologist noted an abnormality and that the area should be examined again by mammography in a few months. Would you be worried or not worried? Now let's supposed that your physician told you that you needed to have an open biopsy of the suspicious area, how worried would you be? While you are waiting for the results of the pathology report, how worried would you be? If your physician told you that the pathologist wanted to send the biopsy out to get a second opinion, how anxious would you be?

Anxiety is a normal reaction. How does anxiety may manifest itself? It manifests itself in denial, tactics to delay diagnosis, feelings of impending death because you were told that you are high risk for breast cancer, sleepless nights, feeling that procedures are extremely painful when they are not and loss of appetite. Once a diagnosis of malignancy is made for primary or recurrent disease how do you cope? Do not be afraid. Many people with a strong prayer life who know God pray and trust in God to see them through. He is with them every step of the way when they call on Him and their fears and anxieties are diminished.

Yes, some people do die from breast cancer, but many are surviving and coping with this disease and staying disease-free for long periods of time. The diagnosis and treatment of breast cancer is one step at a time. There are many women who have walked this path before you and many are willing to discuss with you how they handled their situation. If you are experiencing sleepless nights that interfere with your waking hours, let you physician know and he can subscribe something to help you sleep at night. The more you know about the disease, the less anxiety you will have.

Depression

Depression is grief and sadness that one experiences over a loss. The depression experienced over cancer is not unlike any other depression. The depth of depression experienced by cancer patients is variable and may be minor to a major depressive disorder, which may last years. The emotional response to cancer is different for each patient. How a patient handles the disruptions in lifestyle, body disfigurement, self-image, financial loss, legal concerns and fears about the future are based on the patient's ability to adapt to those changes. The best way to cope with the loss of a breast or ideas that you are no longer beautiful or that you cannot function or that you are going to die is to be actively involved in your treatment decisions and in your daily routines. Do not decide that just because you are undergoing cancer treatment that you cannot work. Discuss your situation with your physician and he will make provisions so that you can maintain an active lifestyle with some limitations. If necessary your physician can refer you to a psychologist or counselor. Try not to let the way you feel cause anxiety within your family. If there are family problems because of your health, discuss these problems openly and directly to relieve the anxiety that family members may be experiencing.

References:

1. Young LS, Fever and septicemia. InRubin RH, Young LS, Clinical Approach to Infection in the Compromised Host. 2nd ed. New York, NY Plenum Medical, 1988, pp 75-114.
2. Cleary JF, Fever and sweats including the immunocompromised hosts. InBerger A, Portenoy RK, Weissman DE, eds.Principles and Practice of Supportive Oncology. Philadelphia, PaLippincott-Raven Publishers, 1998, pp 119-131.
3. Frazier AL; Ryan CT; Rockett H; Willett WC; Colditz GA Division of Pediatric Oncology, Dana-Farber Cancer Institute, Harvard Medical School, Boston,Massachusetts,USA. Lindsay.frazier@channing.harvard.edu. Breast Cancer Res. 2003; 5(3)R59-64 <lindsay.frazier@channing.harvard.edu>.
4. The Institute of Medicine (IOM), part of the National Academy of Sciences, has published a report assessing the scientific knowledge of health effects and possible medical uses of marijuana. The IOM project was funded by the White House Office of National Drug Control Policy. The IOM released its report on March 17, 1999.
5. Breast Cancer Res. 2006; 8:R11
6. Hyde Riley E; Inui TS, et al.Differential association of modifiable health behaviors with hot flashes in perimenopausal and postmenopausal women, J Gen Intern Med. 2004; 19(7)740-6.
7. Kopin IJ, Blombery P, Ebert MH, et al. Disposition and metabolism of MHPG-CD3 in human plasma MHPG as the principal pathway of norepinephrine metabolism and as an important determinant in CSF levels of MHPG. InUsdin E, et al, eds. Frontiers in Biochemical and Pharmacological Research in Depression. New York Raven Press; 1984. 57-68
8. Freedman RR. Core body temperature variation in symptomatic and asymptomatic postmenopausal women brief report.
9. Menopause 2002NIH Consensus and State-of-the-Science

Statements, Volume 22, Number 1, p. 17, March 21–23, 2005; 9:399-401

10. Barton DL, et al "Phase III, placebo-controlled trial of three doses of citalopram for the treatment of hot flashes: NCCTG Trial N05C9" *J Clin Oncol* 2010; DOI: 10.1200/JCO.2009.26.6379.

11. Young T, Rabago D, Zgierska A, Austin D, Finn L. Objective and subjective sleep quality in premenopausal, perimenopausal, and postmenopausal women in the Wisconsin cohort study. Sleep 2003; 26:667-672

12. NIH Consensus and State-of-the-Science Statements, Volume 22, Number 1, p. 17, March 21–23, 2005
Ohayon, M. Archives of Internal Medicine, June 26, 2006; vol 166pp 1262-1268. News release, JAMA/Archives 1.

13. Clarke R, Hilakivi-Clarke L, Cho E, et al. Estrogens, phytoestrogens, and breast cancer. In American Institute for Cancer Research, ed. Dietary phytochemicals in cancer prevention and treatment. New York Plenum Press, 1996:63-85.

14. Bioidentical Hormones for Menopausal Hormone Therapy: Variation on a Theme, Fugh-Berman, A. et Bythrow, J. MS, J Gen Intern Med. 2007 July; 22(7): 1030–1034.

15. Stearns V, Beebe KL, Iyengar M, Dube E. Paroxetine controlled release in the treatment of menopausal hot flashes a randomized controlled trial. JAMA 2003; 289:2827-2834.

16. Cancer Control 6(2)191-197, 1999. 199H. Lee Moffitt Cancer Center and Research Institute, Inc.

17. Smith TJ, Coyne PJ, Staats PS, et al. Implantable drug delivery systems (IDDS) provide sustained pain control, less drug toxicity, and better survival compared to comprehensive medical management (CMM). Program and abstracts of the American Society of Clinical Oncology 39th Annual Meeting; May 31-June 3, 2003; Chicago, Illinois. Abstract 2967.

18. Syrjala KL, Donaldson GW, Davis MW, et al. Relaxation and imagery and cognitive-behavioral training reduces pain during cancer treatment a controlled clinical trial. Pain. 1995; 63:189-198.

19. DeCharms RC, Maeda F, Glover GH, et al. Control over brain activation and pain learned by using real-time functional MRI. Proc Natl Acad Sci 2005; 102:18626-18631

REDUCING BREAST CANCER RISK AND RECURRENCE
THROUGH NUTRITION AND EXERCISE

Nutritional support and diet needs are important during the treatment of breast cancer. The right nutrition helps you to deal with the side effects of treatment and gives you enough caloric intake to replace healthy cells that were destroyed by the treatment. Your physician may consult a registered dietitian to help you with your nutrition needs especially if you are having difficulty in maintaining your weight. [1] Nutrition is also important in reducing the risk of breast cancer and its recurrence. There is very little information given about the dietary habits of women who have survived breast cancer and how it has affected their quality of life. However, it has been established that women who have a diet with higher consumption of eggs, vegetable fat and fiber have a lower risk of breast cancer. It is also known that women who consume more butter and animal fat have an increased risk of breast cancer. [2]

Nutrition

Breast cancer occurs 10 times more in the United States than it does in Asia and Africa. Our Western lifestyle and diet have everything to do with the reasons why breast cancer is so prevalent in our society when compared with others. We live highly sedentary lifestyles and do not exercise. We prefer to eat out rather than cook at home and have control over what we consume. Most of our calories are obtained from fat and sugar. The content of our diet has less than half of the fiber we need. We prefer to eat fried foods, processed foods and sugar. We do not eat enough fresh fruit and vegetables and when we attempt to make changes and buy fresh fruit and vegetables, so often many of us let the fresh fruit and vegetables sit and spoil in our refrigerators.

It is difficult to ascertain the exact role that environmental factors and the exposure to carcinogens (substances that cause cancer) may play in the etiologic role and the development of breast cancer. Dietary factors in the development of cancer are very difficult to study, but evidence does suggest that in certain stages of a woman's life, namely in the stage before birth in the womb and the stage after menopause, diets that induce or cause high estrogen levels do seem to increase the likelihood that a woman will get breast cancer. High levels of estrogen during childhood however, tend to have a protective role against breast cancer.

Dr. Hilakivi-Clarke conducted a study of the offspring of rats on a high fatty diet and of rats that received an injection of genistein, an isoflavone and antioxidant or agent that counteracts damage in the body. Offspring of rats that were fed soy diets showed no increase breast cancer risk and were similar to the offspring of the normal rat population. [3] Offspring of the rats on the high fatty diet that received genistein showed an increase risk of breast cancer.

Evidence suggests that high fat intake, increased red meat and increased animal fat consumption with decreased consumption of fruits and vegetables may increase the risk of breast cancer development. It also appears that the risk of breast cancer may be affected by what happened before you were born and may be based on what your mother ate during her pregnancy, and on what you ate as a child and what you are eating as an adult. **We are what we eat!** Although you cannot change what your mother ate while you were in the womb and what you ate as a child, you can however, make life- style changes in your diet now.

Many women during and after their treatment for breast cancer have a significant weight gain. Given the knowledge that breast cancer rates are increased in patients with a fatty diet, it would behoove women with breast cancer and women who are at an increased risk for breast cancer to make some lifestyle alterations in diet to decrease the risk of breast cancer and the risk of recurrence or the development of a second primary breast cancer. In order to reduce your breast cancer risk you must control your total caloric intake and limit the amount of fat in your diet to less than 30% of your total caloric intake and increase the amount of fresh fruits and vegetables in your diet. Researchers in Toronto, Canada at the National Cancer Institute while studying the dietary habits of women with prior breast cancer found that the risk of dying from breast cancer increases by 50% for every 5% increase in the intake of saturated fat. [4]

The Women's Healthy Eating and Living (WHEL) Diet and the National Cancer Institute diet (NCI) study diets which are rich in plant based foods are represented in the Table 25-1. The WHEL study increased the amount of carotenoids (the beta, alpha and gamma carotenes Vitamin A) in the diet while the NCI study did not. The results of the study

Table 25-1.

	WHEL DIET	NCI DIET
Vegetable servings	5	3
Vegetable juice	16 oz.	0
Fruit Servings	3	2
Fiber (grams)	30	20
% calories from fat	20	<30 [6]

showed breast cancer relapses occurred in only 200 of the 3000 women enrolled in the study.

What we do know about diet and breast cancer prevention comes from the study by Schuster. Schuster's study clearly shows that approximately 9.8% of women with early stage breast cancer when placed on a low-fat diet experienced tumor recurrence, while there was a 12.4% recurrence in patients on a standard diet. [7] The Women's Health Initiative or WHEL diet study of 19,541 postmenopausal women without a previous history of breast cancer showed a greater risk reduction of breast cancer for women on a low fat diet than for women who had a high-fat diet. However, women who had a low fat diet and continued a low fat diet showed no changes is risk reduction. The validity of the study is in question since it relied on the participants self-monitoring and self-reporting of what they had eaten. This was not a controlled study. However, based on the findings of the study it still behooves the women at risk for breast cancer and breast cancer recurrence to consider modifications to the diet that reduce the dietary fat and to increase fruit, vegetables and fiber intake. These modifications in diet are small and easy to make. You can achieve success and maintain good nutrition without starving to death. It's a matter of choice. Here are a few choices or wise decisions you can make to help you in reducing your dietary fat intake:

1) **If you eat on the run or eat out most of the time, start eating out less. Limit the times you eat out to once or twice a week.**
2) **If you can't cook, learn how to cook for yourself. Cooking for yourself can help you make healthy decisions for yourself.**

Most fast food and chain restaurants use saturated or hydrogenated soybean oil to fry French fries, tator tots, fish, chicken, and hamburgers. Soybean oil when heated to high temperatures results in oxidation of the fat and the forming of free radicals that damage cells in the body. Toxic trans-fatty acids clog arteries and are linked to cancer. If you go to an upscale restaurant and have butter with your shrimp and lobster, the butter is usually butter flavored hydrogenated soybean oil. I challenge you to try to find something on the menu that does not have hydrogenated soybean oil in it. It is a so-called natural preservative and gives food a longer shelf life. A longer shelf life means dollar savings and profit to chain restaurants. The presence of hydrogenated fats and soybean oil in the majority of foodstuffs means a high fat diet to you. Breast cancer risk is increased when cooking with hydrogenated fats or vegetable oils rich in linoleic acid. Breast cancer risk is lower for oils rich in oleic acid, i.e. olive and canola oil. [11]

3) Learn how to shop for your groceries. Read labels on what you buy and intend to eat. Stay away from processed foods and meals in a box or meal helpers and processed meats.
4) Buy whole foods and do not eat anything with artificial or synthetic or with natural man-made ingredients or flavors.
Artificial and synthetic food additives have no nutritional value. Some of these additives may be the cause of health problems. If you are plague by sinusitis, start looking the ingredients of what you are eating. If you eliminate everything that says natural flavorings or soybean oil in your diet, you can substantially decrease the percentage of fat in your diet. Soy bean oil and/or its derivatives is an ingredient in 98% of prepared food, sauces, packaged food, salad dressings, soups and broths, cheeses, breads and cakes, chips and dips, the shiny waxy coating on apples and other fresh fruit and some vegetables. Some frozen foods and meats may be dipped in soy before freezing to seal in freshness and increase shelf life. Soybean oil is present in ice cream and dressings, soups and broths, cheeses, breads and cakes, chips and dips, the shiny waxy coating on apples and other fresh fruit and

some vegetables. Some frozen foods and meats may be dipped in soy before freezing to seal in freshness and increase shelf life. Soybean oil is present in ice cream and even injected into meats to make the cut of meat cook and brown evenly and to add flavor. It doesn't take a rocket scientist to know that a little bit of soybean oil in every prepared food item is extra fat grams that are not needed.

5) **Increase the amount of fresh fruits and vegetables in your diet.** Learn how to pick the choicest fruits and vegetables for your consumption. You can get all the vitamins and essential nutrients that you need by eating fresh produce and not processed vegetables and fruits. There is no need to spend money for expensive supplements if you learn how to choose wisely in the grocery store. You will even find that you can save money by not buying processed foods.

Researchers in Montreal, Canada have shown that **diets rich in carotenoids and fish oils may reduce breast cancer risk.** [8] Studies from researchers at New York University School of Medicine have shown a clear benefit of carotenoids in 270 women diagnosed with breast cancer. Patients with low beta-carotene levels had twice the incidence of breast cancer than women with high levels of beta-carotene. [9] Studies in countries with high intake of **omega-3 acids** from fish have lower breast cancer rates. British medical researchers have reported that a high fish oil intake has a protective effect against breast cancer. [10] Among postmenopausal women with a high intake of carotenoids and fish oils the risk of breast cancer is cut in half. **Researchers advocate that a diet with a high content of fruits, carotenoid-rich vegetables, and docosahexaenoic acid (DHA)-rich fish may reduce the risk of breast cancer.** [12]

Researchers from the Harvard School of Public Health found in a study of 32,826 women that women with the high blood levels of folate greater than 14 ng/mL had a 27% lower risk of breast cancer than did women with levels of folate less than 6.4 ng/mL. High levels of vitamin B6, greater than 95.3 pmol/mL were associated with a 30% risk reduction of breast cancer. It can be concluded that diets, which are rich in folate and vitamin B6, may reduce the risk of breast cancer. [13]

It is believed that folate, folic acid exerts a protective effect by preventing errors in DNA replication by helping to regenerate methionine, an amino acid that is a vital component in DNA synthesis. The Shanghai Breast Cancer Study during 1996-1998 found that the dietary intake of 345 micrograms or more of folate daily had a 38% lower risk for the development of breast cancer than in women who had an intake of less than 195 micrograms daily. [14,15] The following foods are high sources for folic acid : asparagus, barley, beef, bran, brewer's yeast, brown rice, cheese, chicken, dates, green leafy vegetables, legumes, lentils, liver, milk, oranges, peas, pork, salmon, tuna, and whole grains. Food sources having the high content of Vitamin B6 are: carrots, chicken, eggs, fish, meat, peas, spinach, sunflower seeds, walnuts, avocados, bananas, beans, broccoli, whole grains, cabbage, cantaloupe, corn, plantains and potatoes.

Phytoestrogens lower breast cancer risks. Isoflavonoids are phytoestrogens. The isoflavonoids, equol and lignan enterolactone, in a case control study of phyto-estrogens, by Ingram et al. lower the risk of developing breast cancer. [17] Bananas are high in anti-oxidants. Eating four to six bananas per week can reduce your cancer risk. Tomatoes, watermelon and pink grapefruit are rich in lycopene. One can of tomato paste has as much lycopene as twenty tomatoes. German research has shown that lycopene reduces the rate of colorectal cancer and the risk of prostate cancer. There has been shown an increase risk of breast cancer in patients who have a family history in which prostate cancer exists. It can't hurt to increase lycopene by the consumption of tomato, watermelon or grapefruit consumption all of which are also rich in Vitamin C. Researchers at the University of Seattle have concluded that Vitamin C may play a crucial role in controlling free radical damage to the DNA in breast tissue and help prevent breast cancer metastases. [18]

Researchers at the National Center of Toxicological Research have found that the antioxidants obtained from the diet, vitamins E and C were effective in protecting against oxidative stress. Manganese superoxide dismutase (MnSOD) is a complex protein that protects the cell's mitochondria or powerhouse from oxidative stress. Some women may have a gene allele or part of a gene that is not as effective in protecting against the oxidative stresses. Researchers found that women who had the less effective MnSOD allele who consumed a diet rich in antioxidants can eliminate their high risk of developing breast cancer. [19]

Olive oil which oleic acid, which has been shown by researchers from Northwestern University's Feinberg School of Medicine to cut the levels of the cancer HER2 gene associated with aggressive breast cancers. Women who consume olive oil more than twice per day are 25% less likely to develop breast cancer than women who use olive oil once per day or less as found in a study conducted by researches at the Athens Medical School and the Harvard School of Public Health. [20]

A Harvard School of Public Health report has shown that legumes may lessen the risk of breast cancer by suppressing the production of enzymes that encourage tumor growth. Women who eat beans twice a week are 24% less likely to develop breast cancer than those who eat beans less often. Women who consume the most dietary calcium (more than 1,250 mg daily) had a 20% lower risk for postmenopausal breast cancer than those with intakes less than 50mg daily. [21] Dietary calcium in the form of three 8-ounce glasses of skim or fat free milk, or an 8-ounce serving of low fat yogurt or 2 to 3-ounce serving of low fat cheese contain the daily requirement of calcium. Calcium and Vitamin D in the form of supplements are not associated with overall lower risk for postmenopausal breast cancer.

Diet Recommendations to Lower Breast Cancer Risk

1) Eat a low-fat high fiber diet with fresh vegetables (broccoli, cabbage, cauliflower, carrots, greens, pumpkin, squash, sweet potatoes or yams). Broccoli, carrots, greens, and cauliflower contain phytoestrogens. Broccoli contains sulphoraphane, which inhibits estrogen binding to tumor cells. Broccoli also contains indol-3 carbinol, a compound that promotes healthy estrogen balance in the body and protects breast cells. Increase your carotenoids by eating two or more servings of dark green, yellow or orange vegetables and fruits daily.

2) Eat more whole grains (brown rice, oats, and wheat).

3) Eat plenty fresh fruits (apples, plums, cherries, apricots, grapefruits, watermelon, grapes, bananas and berries). All fruits and vegetables are high in Vitamin C and anti-oxidants.

4) Eat legumes, peas, lentils and beans at least twice a week to increase your dietary calcium, fiber and genistein (isoflavinoids). Kidney beans, navy beans, pinto beans and black-eyed peas are high in fiber and contain protective phytoestrogens.

5)   Eat plenty tomatoes, tomato sauces, tomato paste, watermelon and pink grapefruits which are lycopene rich.

6) Eat fresh onions and garlic. Peppers, berries, carrots and tomatoes that contain flavinoids. Consider adding more hot red peppers and chili peppers in your diet. [22] They contain cayenne or capsaicin, which aid in the prevention of some cancers and have been found to act as an appetite suppressant for weight reduction and boost metabolism.

7) Eat fish, flaxseed and olive which contain omega3 fatty acids. Canned salmon or tuna fish are options if fresh (not farmed) salmon or tuna cannot be obtained. Fish oil supplements are also acceptable sources for omega3 fatty acids and have been shown to impede breast tumor growth.

8) Limit your intake of red meat. In a study conducted by Harvard it was found that the adolescence period was a period of increased susceptibility to breast cancer. Red meat consumption in early adult life has been associated with breast cancer. [23] This is probably due to the fact that exogenous hormones are used to stimulate the growth of cattle in the United States. The hormones that are given to cattle are present in residual amounts in the consumed meat and have effects on human health.

9) Do not consume any meat, poultry or dairy from animals that have been given hormones. If an animal receives hormones, those same hormones may increase your breast cancer risk.

10) Limit your intake of charred fatty meats and fried foods.

11) Do not eat meat that has been loaded or injected with preservatives.

12) Drink plenty of spring water and limit tap water.

13) Limit your alcohol consumption.

14) Limit alcohol consumption to 4 servings of alcohol per week and no more than 1 serving per day. When more than one drink is consumed at one time, the risk of breast cancer increases. If you must drink, the consumption of red wine is a good choice because it contains antioxidants. Alcohol is associated with increased breast cancer risk and risk of recurrence for ER + breast tumors. [24] Women who consume alcohol within 5 years before the diagnosis of breast cancer appear to have an improved survival not attributable to differences in screening, treatment and stage of disease.[25]

15) Drink fruit and vegetable drinks that are fresh and homemade.

16) Drink low fat or skim milk and low-fat cottage cheese and cheeses, low-fat yogurt or ice cream. These milk products are rich in Vitamin D and calcium.

17) Limit the amount of carbohydrates and refined sugars and processed foods in your diet.

18) Read labels and limit the amount of natural and artificial preservatives.

19) Eat at home more often and prepare your own food.

Table 25-2.

DIET TO LOWER BREAST CANCER RISK AND RECURRENCE		
FOOD TYPE	SERVINGS/DAY	YOUR CHOICES
FRUIT	2-3	Bananas (4 - 6/week), tomatoes or tomato paste, peaches, watermelons, cantaloupes, grapefruit, apples, pears, plums, cherries, apricots, oranges, berries, dates, fresh fruit drinks
VEGETABLES	3-5	Broccoli, cabbage, cauliflower, brussel sprouts, asparagus, spinach, dark greens, asparagus, carrots, sweet potatoes (yams) pumpkin, squash, legumes, peas, lentils, beans(>2servings/week); potatoes, green peppers, hot red and chili peppers, cayenne pepper, fresh onions and garlic, fresh vegetable juice (16 oz)
FIBER	20-30 GRAMS	Diet high in vegetables and fruits as above, whole grain breads, cereals, grain, brown rice, barley
% CALORIES FAT	20-30	Olive oil (twice daily), Fresh or canned (not farmed) salmon, tuna or mackerel, fish oil supplements, hormone free meat poultry and dairy (3 -8 oz glasses of low or fat free milk, 8 oz low fat yogurt, or 3 oz cheese), eggs

Exercise

It is common knowledge that obesity has been linked to numerous cancers and most notably breast cancer. Obesity or being overweight occurs when a high amount of calories are consumed and there is limited physical inactivity. If you are overweight it is important to determine the reason for being overweight. Your doctor can determine if your obesity is because of lack of physical activity or due to an endocrine or gland problem. Before increasing your physical activity or placing yourself on a diet you should consult your doctor first.

By increasing your physical activity you can modify your risks for breast cancer and have protection from breast cancer recurrence as well as protection against other malignancies. Women who have been previously diagnosed with in situ or invasive ductal carcinoma and participate in one to three hours of physical activity per week have a 30% lower risk of breast cancer recurrence. [5] Acceptable exercise could be any of the following: aerobic exercise classes, swimming, gymnastics, gym workouts, free weights, running or jogging and walking. Just increasing physical activity to house cleaning twice a week has been shown to decrease breast cancer risk by 20%. I am not advocating for you to follow a specific diet or exercise program. Just the two words, diet and exercise seem to have negative connotations for many in this society. I am however, recommending lifestyle modifications that you can make which should be easy to do, just simple methods to increase you physical activity, especially if you have been sedentary most of your life.

I prefer working out three times a week doing aerobic training for thirty minutes in the form of cycling with a standard or reclined bicycle or running with an inclined treadmill three times a week for thirty minutes followed by thirty minutes of high repetition sets (15 to 20 reps) using light weights. This is an excellent cardiovascular workout which burns up any excess calories that I may have consumed and helps maintain adequate muscle mass, maintain an adequate amount of body fat and strengthens bones.

This type of exercise is not something that you can automatically do if you are sedentary. You have to begin exercising slowly and build up your endurance slowly. If you are not physically, you can start by riding an exercise bike for 5 minutes daily for a week then increasing the minutes over time. You can start out working with weights similarly. If you are overweight this process may be slower, you may have to start by walking and then later start an aerobic program. The key is to start a program and to build up muscle mass while eating the right type and amount of food that your body needs. You have to eat to build muscle, but do not eat high caloric high fat snacks, substitute fruits instead. Make sure that you eat at least three meals a day and supply your body with the energy it needs so that the muscles that you do have do not begin to deteriorate or breakdown because of lack of food. You should eat so that you can build up your muscle cells. Do not begin an exercise program until you have first consulted your physician.

References:

1. Massie MJ, Holland JC. Overview of normal reactions and prevalence of psychiatric disorders. Holland JC, Rowland JH, eds Handbook of Psychooncology Psychological Care of the Patient With Cancer. New York, NY Oxford University Press, 1989, pp 273-82.
2. Desiree Lie, MD, MSEd, Clinical Professor of Family Medicine; Director, Division of Faculty Development, University of California, Irvine School of Medicine, Irvine, California. Medscape Medical News 2005. 2005 Medscape.
3. Prenatal, Childhood Diets May Play Most Important Role in Breast Cancer Risk Medscape Medical News 2000.
4. Jain, Meera, et al. Premorbid diet and the prognosis of women with breast cancer. Journal of the National Cancer Institute, Vol. 86, No. 18, September 21, 1994, pp. 1390-97.
5. Bernstein, Leslie, et al. Physical exercise and reduced risk of breast cancer in young women. Journal of the National Cancer Institute, Vol. 86, No. 18, September 21, 1994, pp. 1403-08
6. Jones VE, Hollenbach K, Rock C, et al. The women's health eating and living (WHEL) study a nutritional intervention study in breast cancer survivors. Program and abstracts of the 23rd Annual San Antonio Breast Cancer Symposium; December 6-9, 2000; San Antonio, Texas. Abstract 154. Breast Cancer Res Treat. 2000, 64:49.

7. Schuster, L., Low-Fat Diet May Cut Risk of Breast Cancer Recurrence Medscape Medical News 2005. 2005 Medscape

8. Nkondjock, A. and Ghadirian, P. Intake of specific carotenoids and essential fatty acids and breast cancer risk in Montreal, Canada. American Journal of Clinical Nutrition, Vol. 79, May 2004, pp. 857-64.

9. Toniolo, Paolo, et al. Serum carotenoids and breast cancer. American Journal of Epidemiology, Vol. 153, June 15, 2001, pp. 1142-51.

10. Caygill, C.P.J., et al. Fat, fish, fish oil and cancer. British Journal of Cancer, Vol. 74, No. 1, July 1996, pp. 159-64

11. Jun Wang, John, E. et al., Dietary Fat, Cooking Fat, and Breast Cancer Risk in a Multiethnic Population , <u>Nutrition and Cancer</u>, Volume <u>60</u>, Issue <u>4</u> July 2008 , pages 492 - 504

12. Bagga, Dilprit, et al. Dietary modulation of omega-3/omega-6 polyunsaturated fatty acid ratios in patients with breast cancer. Journal of the National Cancer Institute, Vol. 89, August 6, 1997, pp. 1123-31.

13. Zhang, SM, et al. Plasma folate, vitamin B6, vitamin B12, homocysteine, and risk of breast cancer. Journal of the National Cancer Institute, Vol. 95, March 5, 2003, pp. 373-80.

14. Shrubsole, Martha J., et al. Dietary folate intake and breast cancer risk results from the Shanghai Breast Cancer Study. Cancer Research, Vol. 61, October 1, 2001, pp. 7136-41.

15. Larsen, HR. International Health News. Summaries of latest research concerning breast cancer prevention.

16. Ingram, David, et al. Case-control study of phyto-estrogens and breast cancer. The Lancet, Vol. 350, October 4, 1997, pp. 990-9415.Messina, Mark, et al. Phyto-estrogens and breast cancer. The Lancet, Vol. 350, October 4, 1997, pp. 971-72 (commentary)

17. Malins, Donald C., et al. Progression of human breast cancers to the metastatic state is linked to hydroxyl radical-induced DNA damage. Proceedings of the National Academy of Sciences USA, Vol. 93, No. 6, March 19, 1996, pp. 2557-63.

18. Ambrosone, Christine B., et al. Manganese superoxide dismutase (MnSOD) genetic polymorphisms, dietary antioxidants, and risk of breast cancer. Cancer Research, Vol. 59, February 1, 1999, pp.

602- 0618. 18.

19. Trichopoulou, Antonia, et al. Consumption of olive oil and specific food groups in relation to breast cancer risk in Greece. Journal of the National Cancer Institute, Vol. 87, No. 2, January 18, 1995, pp. 110-16

20. Cancer Epidemiology Biomarker Prevent. 200514:2898-2904.

21. Balch, Phyllis A. Prescription for herbal healing. Penguin Putnam, Inc, 2002. p 43-44.

23. Linos, Fleni, et al. , Red Meat Consumption during Adolescence among Premenopausal Women and Risk of Breast Cancer, Cancer Epidemiol Biomarkers Prev 2008;17(8):2146–51.

24. Deandrea, Silcia, Talamini R. et al., Alcohol and Breast Cancer Risk Defined by Estrogen and Progesterone Receptor Status: A Case-Control Study, Cancer Epidemiol Biomarkers Prev 2008;17(8):2025–8.

25. Reding, Kerryn, Daling JR et al., Effect of Prediagnostic Alcohol

26. Consumption on Survival after Breast Cancer in Young Women, Cancer Epidemiol Biomarkers Prev 2008;17(8):1988–96.

Lessons To Be Learned

1) Reduce the amount of dietary fat you consume.
2) If you are overweight, increase your physical activity.
3) Increase your consumption of fresh fruits and vegetables.
4) Increase the amount of fiber in your diet.
5) Limit your alcohol intake.
6) Begin a regular exercise program after consulting your doctor.

SURVIVORSHIP AND LIFE AFTER BREAST CANCER

The good news is that there is life after breast cancer. The quality of life is dependent upon how well the adverse effects of having cancer are minimized. Survivorship depends on whether or not your physical, psychological, social and spiritual needs and concerns are addressed. Most cancer patients experience emotional difficulty of some type. Many patients with breast cancer will adjust normally, but some may experience adjustment disorders and some significant mental disorders in which a physician may need to intervene and prescribe medication to help the patient adjust during this time of difficulty.

Once breast cancer has been diagnosed and successfully treated, survivorship depends on continued surveillance. This means routine close follow-up as recommended by your physician. You do not have the option increasing the length of time between the follow-up examinations by your healthcare provider and your annual mammography visits. Do not make excuses or procrastinate. Make sure you tell your physician how you have been feeling. If you have any question concerning an anti-estrogen that you may be taking ask those questions. Convey to your physician your feelings and any concerns that you may have. If you have questions on how you are to take care of yourself don't be afraid to ask them. If your physician orders some additional scans or laboratory tests, make sure that you get the tests done. Your physician is not requesting these tests for your treatment and not for curiosity, it is for your health. These tests are imperative for your follow-up care.

The diagnosis of breast cancer not only impacts the patient's physical health, but as I alluded to it also has a mental and emotional impact, which varies with each patient. It also impacts the family and especially the spouse who may invariably feel like he is somewhat neglected in the treatment process. The spouse is expected to be available emotionally and physically as a support to the cancer patient at home where duties of the household may have shifted, clinic appointments and meetings may place additional demands on the spouse. Spouses try hard to maintain normality amidst the uncertainty in their lives and the life of their wife. The spouse may not even be asked how they are coping. Most men tend to be silent about their spouse's illness. They tend to suppress their true emotions and how they are feeling about the entire treatment plan. Invariably their sexual and physical needs have been put on the back burner. They wonder about the fragility of their partner and wonder whether or not the spouse will have any sexual desire ever again.

I did not find out my spouse's true feelings and thought until three years post treatment. In his family's culture the wife is supposed to survive the husband. If a wife dies then it reflects badly upon the husband and the opinion is that he did not take care of his wife. His culture also does not speak openly about illnesses and death. That is the reason why he did not want me to tell my siblings and other family members about my illness, but I vehemently disagreed. My husband also told me that he was afraid that he was going to lose me. He said that when he saw the mass that came from underneath my arm and looked at the slide that I had prepared and when I told him that it was breast cancer, he said that he died. Several physicians offered to speak with him but he declined any help. Your health care professionals should be able to address thia type of difficulties.
l

Family members and friends can be a tremendous support at this time. The following is my opinion on how a person with breast cancer should be approached:

- Do not offer any more support than what the individual asks. If you are needed the patient or the patients spouse or doctor will let you know. The amount of support that is needed varies between patients just like manner of physically and emotionally adjustment between patients.

-Do not make the individual feel helpless. Many patients already feel sad and worried, because they don't know what to expect in the present or in the future, whether or not they will die of cancer or if the cancer will come back after they are treated. Patients going through chemotherapy may be extremely, but many want to do things for themselves and want to function as normally as they can, even if it takes two hours to do something that may normally have taken the individual fifteen minutes to do.

-Do not be weepy and sorrowful when you visit the individual. Note that the individual is not dead yet and the patient does not need you to close and seal the casket. Note that this individual needs at this time is a positive feeling and spirit and hope from you

and not negativity.
- Do not tell the individual that you understand unless you have been through the exact same thing.
- If you are needed you will be told directly by the doctor or the individual.

If you are the one being treated:

> - Have children try to educate them on what is happening and what physical changes they may notice. Tell them that they can ask their parent(s) about any concern or questions that they may have.
> - Try to keep your children's daily routine unchanged.

References:

1. Harrow, Alison, Wells, Mary et al. Ambiguity and uncertainty: The ongoing concerns of male partners of women treated for breast cancer. School of Nursing and Midwifery, University of Dundee, 11 Airlie Place, Dundee, DD1 4HJ Scotland, UK RCN Scotland, 42 South Oswald Road, Edinburgh, EH9 2HH Scotland, UK . June 10, 2008.

The most important goal of cancer treatment is stop the spread of the cancer and to help the patient return to good health and improve the patient's quality of life. Complementary and alternative medical treatments (CAM) may include the following:
- psychological support
- group therapy and cancer support groups
- nutritional supplements
- vitamins or herbs
- acupuncture
- massage, relaxation and yoga
- exercise
- psychic healing
- use of toxic substances (i.e. laetrile)

If you are considering using complementary and alternative medicine do not begin such therapies until you have sought the advice of your oncologist or regular physician. Many complementary and alternative medicine therapies go against the grain of conventional medicine. The effectiveness of the therapies must be studied using the scientific methods and proven by data for the effectiveness of such treatments. Some CAM can improve the effectiveness of conventional treatment, but your physician must be informed of the treatment you may be receiving since some treatments may adversely effect your conventional treatment. It is important that you make sure that your physician is aware of any alternative nutriments, supplements, herbal, detox procedures, frequency, energy or magnetic therapies, oxygen therapy or any other treatments that you may purchase or seek from other practitioners.

Do not commit to CAM without conventional therapy. CAM therapies do not cure cancer. Use some common sense. Rubbing wormwood oil or vitamin E oil over your breast cannot remove the cancer. Cancers are not caused by parasites and cancer cells can live in a high oxygen environment. Laetrile is toxic and does not cure cancer. It is cyanide and can kill a patient. CAM therapies should be used as adjunctive treatment to your conventional treatment plan and used only after consulting you physician. Your physician is probably more knowledgeable about such treatments than you think and will make every effort to understand your needs so that an effective treatment plan can be developed and tailored just for you and so that your progress can be monitored.

Psychological treatment and support

I mentioned previously that when a patient is given the diagnosis of cancer, there is an adjustment period and it is different for each patient. Some patients may not adjust and may go into severe depression and this need to be treated. Your physician is aware of this if you need treatment your physician will prescribe treatment. If your physician feels that considerable support is needed, a psychiatrist or psychologist may be consulted. Some psychologists may use mind-body therapy, using either hypnosis or biofeedback to promote greater emotional and spiritual well-being. This may also include massage therapy, meditation, music therapy, yoga, other exercises and imagery techniques.

Breast Cancer Support Groups

There are numerous **support groups** for patients with cancer, local and online. The following is a short list:

- American Cancer Society - Call you local society for a list of support groups
- Susan G. Komen Foundation- http://www.komen.org Research, education, screening and treatment and numerous affiliates
- Breast Cancer Support- http://www.bcsupport.org The site has a meeting place for survivors and is a source for information on breast cancer treatment and recurrence, as well as grief support.
- Caring 4 Cancer- http://www.cancer4caring.com This site offer support for all cancer groups, with information and an electronic health record and messaging.
- WAR Program -http://www.breastmd.org/war_support.html Women At Risk Program support group sponsored by Columbia University
-BreastCancer2
http://health.groups.yahoo.com/group/breastcancer2
-Breast Cancer
- Breast Cancer Support Group on the Web over 170members
-Young Breast Cancer Survivors -692 members with shared

experiences and educational posts http://health.groups.yahoo.com/ group/youngbreastcancersurvivors/
- BreastCancerCare(SECA)-Secondary breast cancer support group Http://www.breastcancercare.org.uk/
-Sisters Network, Inc.Http://www.webmd.com/hw/breast_cancer/
National African American breast cancer survivors organization.
-Community Cancer Support Project. Stanford University.
Http://www.stanford.edu/dept/PBS/CCSP/

Nutritional Approaches and Supplements
Vitamins and Herbal Therapies

CAM offers nutritional approaches using macrobiotics and special diets for cancer patients. The approach focuses on nutritional healing. This appears to be a sound and very popular therapy. It focuses on prevention and possibly cures for a cancer by decreasing cancer risks with a low-fat high-fiber diet with plenty of fresh fruits, vegetables and whole grains. There are three main diets, wheat grass with raw foods, macrobiotic (traditional Japanese) with whole grains and vegetables, and the Moerman regimen, which is a meatless high-fiber diet, which includes supplements. A U.S. Women's Health Initiative study in 2009 found that there was no link between multivitamin use and the likelihood of developing breast cancer. A Puerto Rican study showed protective effects against breast cancer and a Swedish study found that older women who used multivitamins were more likely that non-users to develop breast cancer.[1] If you are considering vitamins to decrease the risk of breast cancer recurrence or the risk of developing breast cancer consider getting vitamins and minerals from the natural food sources in a well balanced diet.

The following nutrients have been used by some women diagnosed with breast cancer to help prevent recurrences or to avoid breast cancer. **Coenzyme Q** has been promoted for use in breast cancer patients to reduce the risk of breast cancer. It is theoretically used to improve cellular oxygen. Coenzyme Q has been shown to reduce heart toxicity from chemotherapy with Doxorubicin in some patients. It is an antioxidant. If you are on blood thinners or anticoagulants, do not take Coenzyme Q for it has been known to interact with the blood thinner Warfarin.

Garlic, zinc, Echinacea, and shark cartilage have been used to boost the immune system by activating certain cells or lymphocyte white blood cells of the immune system, the T helper cells, natural killer cells and B- cells. Shark cartilage may have some anti-inflammatory properties, but claims that it has any anti-cancer benefits have not been supported in human trials. Fish oil, **omega-3-fatty acid** consumption has been linked to a decrease in invasive ductal carcinoma of the breast, but further investigation is needed. **Multivitamin complexes with calcium, magnesium, potassium and zinc** have been used for balance nutrition commonly by half of Americans. A Swedish study recently linked the association between multivitamin use and breast cancer stating that there was an 18% increased risk of breast cancer with multivitamin use.[2] Zinc and magnesium have no proven effect as anti-cancer treatments. Some women take natural **beta-carotene or carotenoids and Vitamin B complex** to improve cellular function and carotene, natural carrot oil is a potent antioxidant that may reduce breast cancer risk. **Vitamins C and E** also have antioxidant activity. Try to avoid the supplements and look for natural dietary sources. It has been shown that **vitamins E and B-6** are associated with a decreased risk for breast cancer. Vitamin C has undergone scrutiny because of a laboratory study stating that it enhanced cancer cell growth, but this result is unclear. **Calcium** provides protection from breast cancer. Cocoa, green tea and grape seed are **polyphenols** and antioxidants. **Alpha lipoic acid (ALA)** has been shown to be a powerful antioxidant also and can be found in red meats, spinach, broccoli and brewer's yeast and has been shown to decrease the likelihood of breast cancer metastases. The compound **superoxide dismutase**, which destroys free radicals, should only be used under physician supervision. **Glutamate with oxidizers** has been used during chemotherapy to prevent nerve damage, numbness of the hands and feet and many oncologists prescribe it routinely.

Laetrile/Vitamin B-17 is a nitriloside and known as the anti-cancer vitamin. It is derived from the kernel of the apricot seed. Use of laetrile is banned in the United States. Deaths have resulted from the use of Laetrile because of the thiocyanate which is produced by the body through the break down or Vitamin B-17. The amount and dosage hard to control and increases the potential for cyanide poisoning. Laetrile became a popular alternative treatment in the 1970s but remains an unproven cancer treatment. In a trial study using Laetrile 90% of patients had progression of their disease. The mean survival of a the patients in the study was 4.8months.[3]

Herbal remedies and various internal and external treatments have been used since ancient times. The purpose of such treatment is to strengthen the body's ability to maintain health or restore health and eliminate cancer cells, but there is no such thing as a cure-all plant. There are no castor oil packs or cleanses that can cure or prevent breast cancer. All herbs have side effects just like medicines and the dosing and standardization and potency of herbs differ. If you are considering drinking herbal teas i.e. ginger, green tea, peppermint and red clover instead of regular tea or using soy or herbal supplements or phytoestrogens my advice to use is to reconsider and the consider with care.

Phytoestrogens are in high content in herbs like red clover, turmeric and black cohosh. It was thought that phytoestrogens may block receptors in breast cancer cells and decrease exposure of these cells to the body's normal estrogens, which are stronger. The diets of Asians are soy-rich and have low levels of genistein and equol. The antiproliferative properties of these phytoestrogens have been documented. It was thought that soy extracts and ginseng may inhibit the growth of breast cancer cells but this may not be the case. There is no direct evidence that herbal medicines can increase or decrease breast cancer risk.

Do not use the following herbs long-term if you have a hormone sensitive Estrogen receptor positive tumor: Black Cohish, Blue cohosh, Chasteberry, Fennel, Dang gui, Dog quai, Ginseng, hop, Motherwort leaf, saw palmetto, Rhodiola rosea, Kudzu, Flaxseed, Licorice, Cordyceps, Red clover, Soy, Vitex berry, Wild yam, Dan Shen and Peony Powder. These herbs have estrogen-like actions and should not be used long-term by women with breast cancer or by women at high risk for breast cancer. The herb, Milk thistle contains a powerful antioxidant Silymarin that is promising in fighting breast cancer.

Acupuncture

Acupuncture is part of Traditional Chinese Medicine. It is a procedure in which thin needles are inserted into points in the skin called acupuncture points. The procedure is not painful when performed correctly. A typical treatment has 6 to 12 needles inserted and lasts from 20 to 60 minutes. Acupuncture is believed to stimulate the nervous system to release natural painkillers and to stimulate cells of the immune system to migrate to the weakened area of the body. Acupuncture has been shown to help relieve fatigue, control hot flashes, lessen nausea and vomiting and pain in women with breast cancer. If you have swelling of your arm or have had the lymph nodes under your arm removed, acupuncture needles should not be inserted into that arm. Make sure if you intend to have acupuncture, that the acupuncturist uses sterile needles that have been cleaned with alcohol or a disinfectant. If your doctor tells you that you have a low white blood cell count or if you have a known bleeding disorder or are taking blood thinners do not use acupuncture.

Massage Therapy

Studies have shown that massage therapy targeting the back, head and neck twice a week helps women cope with breast cancer. The women in the study experienced less anxiety and pain following the massage. Researches found the dopamine levels of the blood and natural killer cells and lymphocytes are also increased with the massage treatments.[4]

Massage therapy is also used for breast cancer related lymphedema. Lymphedema is swelling of the arm and/or trunk of the breast cancer patient after surgery and radiation therapy. Lymphedema is a direct complication of surgery and some edema or swelling may occur in up to 25% of breast cancer patients.[5,6] Manual lymphatic drainage techniques by a specialized compression wraps, skin care and exercise help to reduce and alleviate the swelling. Women with breast cancer may receive treatments by specialized therapists employing manual lymphatic drainage (MLD) or be taught a simple lymphatic drainage (SLD) method by an experienced MLD therapist.

If you consult an MLD therapist make sure that you have written information, drawings and/or a video to supplement the teaching of the therapist. Make sure you find time to fit SLD into your lifestyle. Compression garments are usually worn when performing SLD. The frequency of treatments may be reduced over time. MLD and SLD should not be performed if there is inflammation of the skin and underlying tissue. It should not be performed if you have heart disease or heart failure. It should not be performed if you have active tuberculosis (TB) or untreated cancer.

Progressive Muscle Relaxation (PMR)

Progressive Muscle Relaxation or PMR is a muscle relation technique used to bring about physical relaxation. The technique is begun by tensing and relaxing the toes of one foot, inhaling when tensing the muscles and exhaling when relaxing the muscles. Each muscle of the one leg is tenses and relaxed then the other leg, progressing to each muscle group in the body. Some studies with breast cancer patients have shown reduction of nausea, vomiting, anxiety and depression using this technique. An occasional patient has experienced increased anxiety, fear, and pain with heart palpitations or irregularities.

Stress Reduction

Stress reduction by using guided imagery exercises and relaxation techniques is another complementary therapy to help a breast cancer patient cope. Certain images, smells, touch, tastes or sounds may give the body a positive message and experience, putting it in a relaxed state. This is the so-called mind/body connection, your mind's perception of what is happening around you. Imagery experienced by the mind can give the body a message to cause physiological change and healing. I have seen some patients request to see their tumor under the microscope, so that they could have an image of what they were fighting. They wanted to use the cellular level imagery so that they could try to direct the cells of their immune system to what they needed to fight.

Exercise

Exercise is imperative no matter what type of surgery you have had, since breast surgery affects your arm. It effects the way you move your arm, how you take a deep breath and all of your movements and your daily activities, be they personal care or chores. Your doctor can suggest a a physical therapist or an occupational therapist that can help you design a special exercise program for you if you do not have full use of your arm 3 weeks after surgery. Exercises can begin after all drains and sutures are removed. Exercises should be directed to improve arm and shoulder strength and increase your range of motion. Exercise is a great benefit to the breast cancer patient. Those who exercise 3 to 5 hours a week can cut the risk of dying from breast cancer by 50% when compared to women with sedentary lifestyles.[7] Sedentary lifestyles lead to obesity which leads to higher insulin and insulin growth factors which promotes the growth of breast cancer.[8] Physical activity decreases the incidence of breast cancer and moderate aerobic exercise decreases insulin levels and insulin-like growth factors thereby decreasing the recurrence of breast cancer and resulting in a better prognosis for the breast cancer patient.[9]

Here are a few simple exercises that can be done the first few days after surgery are:
- While lying down slightly raise the affected arm above your chest for 45 minutes. Do at least twice a day. Use pillows and make sure that your hand is higher than your wrist and your elbow higher than your shoulder. This will help decrease the amount of swelling after surgery.
- While your arm is raised open and close your hand 20 times, then bend your elbow repeat five times. This contracts the muscles of the arm and helps pump the lymph fluid in out of your arm.
- Practice deep breathing using slow breaths while lying down and breathe in as much air as you can by pushing your belly button out and then breathing out and relaxing. Repeat this at least 5 times.

It is normal to experience some numbness and tingling and soreness of the back of the arm after surgery. Surgery irritates and pulls the nerves. It is not unusual for you to experience tightness of the arm and armpit. Within a week after surgery you can begin these stretching exercises. Wear loose clothes while doing these exercises. Do them at least 7 times.

These exercise should be done with you lying flat on your back on the floor or in the bead with your knees and hip bent. Do not wear anything that would restrict your stretching.

- Place a broomstick in the palms of your hands then lift the stick over your head as far as you can and continue to lift until you feel the stretch in your affected arm and hold for 5 seconds. Repeat 7 times.
- Clasp your hand behind your neck with elbows pointing up. Move your elbows apart and down to the floor or bed. Repeat the sequence 7 times.

Do these exercises while sitting up in a chair with your back against the chair close to a table:

- Place your unaffected arm palm down then place the affected arm on the table with your elbow straight. Slowly slide the affected arm forward to the opposite side of the table until you feel your shoulder blade move. Repeat the sequence 7 times.
- While sitting in a chair in front of a mirror with your elbows bent and both arms to your side, bring your elbows together behind you, squeezing your shoulder blades. Keep your shoulders level while doing this exercise. Repeat the sequence 7 times.

This side bend exercise helps your trunk movement:

- While sitting in a chair clasp your hands in front of you and lift your arms over your head and straighten your arms. With your arms over your head bend your trunk to the right keeping your arms overhead. Repeat the same sequence bending to the left, then repeat 7 times.

These exercises are to be done while standing:
- While standing facing a corner with toes 8 inches from the corner, bend your elbows at shoulder height and put your forearms on the wall, one on one side of the corner and the other on the other side of the corner. Keeping your arms and feet in place move your chest towards the corner until you feel a stretch across your chest and shoulders. Repeat sequence 7 times.

If you feel weak or loose your balance stop the exercises. Cease or stop the exercises if you feel heaviness in your arm or the swelling increases or if you feel light headed have blurred vision or experience unusual numbness or tingling.

Yoga

Yoga is a ancient technique from India Sanskrit meaning "union" and referring to the body, mind and soul. It involves sitting and stretching the body into different poses and postures called Asana. It can also include breathing, chanting, meditation and inspirational reading. If you are a Christian and are considering the benefits of yoga, I urge you to seek an instructor who teaches the exercises but does not use chanting, meditation and inspirational reading and affirmation statements. Hinduism considers Man and GOD as One in other words man is GOD.[10]   In Hinduism, the ideas of a personal, loving GOD are rejected. Do not align yourself with these false teachings. GOD is the Creator and we are look to God for our salvation. The world is not an illusion, it is GOD's creation. Beware of the New Spirituality.

Breast cancer patients who participate in yoga exercises tend to have better health, less fatigue and sleepiness and a sense of well being and an improved quality of life.[11] Exercises particularly of value to the breast cancer patient is the balanced freedom of movement of the shoulder blade, collarbone and head or top of the humerus bone of the upper arm. The following poses are effective:

- Upward Salute
- Upward Prayer Position

- Prayer Position behind the back)
- Cow Face Position
- Eagle Position
- Extended Child's Pose
- Mountain Pose
- Wide legged Standing Forward Bend
- Triangle Pose
- Upward Bow Pose
- Two-Legged Inverted Staff Pose

Biotherapy/ Immunotherapy

Biotherapy is biological therapy or immunotherapy which is a treatment that works with the immune system to help fight cancer by slowing or stopping the growth of cancer cells and helping the immune system destroy or remove cancer cells by impeding or stopping the spread of cancer cells to other parts of the body. The immune system consists of the following parts in the body: the lymph nodes, tonsils, spleen, bone marrow, thymus gland and five types of white blood cells. The cells that make up the immune system are monocytes (a type of white blood cell), T and B lymphocytes and Natural killer cells.

Biotherapy is a form of cancer vaccine that helps the body fight cancer by aiding the immune system. The biotherapy vaccine used for breast cancer is Herceptin or Trastuzumab used to treat breast cancers with HER2+ overexpression. Besides using vaccines, interferon may be used to stop cells from dividing. Interleukins (IL) are proteins that help coordinate the cells of the immune system so that they can distinguish and fight cancer cells. Monoclonal (a single clone) antibodies target certain proteins on the cancer cells and are effective in certain types of breast cancer. Gene therapy is a promising therapy to correct gene mutations.

Immunologic therapies are based on the fact that cancer occurs because of a defect in the body's immune system. It is hoped that by **immunotherapy** the body can be tricked into producing antibodies to fight breast cancer cells. Unfortunately for reasons unknown, immunotherapy has been ineffective in the majority of cancers including breast cancer.[12] Researchers are trying to develop a molecules that will trigger the production of antibodies to one of the carbohydrate antigens or sites on a breast cancer cell that are capable of producing an immune response. Researchers have found that the complex IL-16 is capable of decreasing the breast cancer tumor burden in a study involving mice. It is hope that a similar immune response will occur when testing humans.

A Mucin1 (MUC1) glycoprotein (carbohydrate protein) was targeted in a large study of breast cancer patients with Stage II disease. Those patients who developed antibodies in the more than 5 year period had no recurrences and those using a placebo had a 27% recurrence rate. This suggests that there may be some benefit for patients receiving MUC1 immunotherapy but an additional phase III trial or study must be done. [13] Other therapies being used are detoxifying therapies with an emphasis on non-toxic or hexagonal water and vitamins. There are pharmacological therapies, which use biologic compounds or pharmaceutical agents directed at re-establishing the immune system. This is based on a theory that a substance excreted by the cancer cells has shut down immune system.

As with any other treatment biotherapy does have its side effects. The side effects may present as flu like symptoms with fevers, chills muscles aches and pains, and fatigue. More serious effects are liver and nerve toxicity, tissue swelling and edema with difficulty breathing and loss of appetite.

Spirituality

The New Age Spirituality with its shift from GOD to humanism has wormed its way into our American society. It entails everything from psychic healing, mediums, astrology, magic and altered trancelike states and so-called Forces. These are simply put occult practices and Christians are not to be defiled by them. Leviticus 19:21 of the Bible states: "Give no regard to mediums and familiar spirits; do not seek after them, to be defiled by them: I am the Lord your GOD."

The practice of **psychic healing** seeks to eliminate the karmic causes of illness that may be causing physical disease. The practice uses a healer who is a channel of Divine energy from the Supreme Being. This practice is also known as Ayurvedic Medicine (used by Chopra) that is practiced in India and similar practices like Reiki, Thai Chi, Yoga, Mind Control and Transcendental Meditation. Psychic surgery originated in the Philipines and in Brazil in the 1950s. The surgeries are performed by crafty psychics who do not use any surgical tools. The surgery is spiritual as well as psychological. The procedure is painless and most psychic surgeons by slight of hand remove blood clots or flesh or foreign material from the patient's body which was the result of an evil spirit possession. The basis of the healings is the healer imagining that he/she is a channel for Divine energy or that God is using them as a channel for positive energy. Channeling is in essence spirit or demon possession and in many cases pure fraud. If you belong to a institutionalized religion or are Christian I urge you to go to your church official and inquire if there are support groups or prayer groups for the sick in your congregation.

Spirituality has a lot to do with whether or not one continues to be preoccupied with negative outlook on the changes of life or whether or not one is able to adapt. If you are irrational in your belief about the disease and as to whether or not you will survive, then your thoughts may affect your ability to adapt and may make your prognosis worse because you have considered your condition hopeless when it may not be. Given two patients with similar age, stage and grade of disease, why does one survive and the other die? Could it be the irrational fears, grief and despair that affect the ability to adapt and survive? Does one patient have supporting family and friends and the other no support? Does one patient believe that GOD can see her through this time in life and the other have no belief in GOD? Spirituality, religion and prayer are important to the quality of life in people diagnosed with cancer. It helps the cancer patient to cope with illness and gives them a sense of well-being, both physically and psychologically and effects the immune system.

If you are experiencing depression, discuss it with your physician. Your physician may recommend counseling for you. If you believed in GOD at one time, but have staggered away from your faith, know that GOD is still there waiting for you and that HE cares and is always there for you even when you feel that no one is. HE still believes in you. Never, never underestimate the power of prayer. If you have friends that are spiritual, ask them to pray for you. If you can't pray, ask your friends to pray with you. No prayer goes unanswered.

The Power of Prayer

The laying of the hands upon the patient, the anointing with oil, prayer and spiritual support is important during this time. Some patients may have shorter recovery periods and even healing from personal and intercessory prayer. I believe in Jesus Christ and His powers of healing and the powers that he bestowed upon his apostles. If you have faith as small as a mustard seed in Jesus Christ and believe that He can heal you of all diseases and infirmities, spiritual and physical, you can be healed through his name. The Gospels of the Bible are full of the stories of Christ's healings:

Matthew 4:2

> *And Jesus went about Galilee, teaching in their synagogues, preaching the gospel of the kingdom, and healing all kinds of sickness and all kinds of disease among the people.*

Matthew 4:24

> *His fame went through all Syria; and they brought to Him all sick people who were afflicted with various diseases and torments, and those who were demoned possessed, epileptics, and paralytics; and He healed them.*

Matthew 8:3

> *Then Jesus put out His hand and touched him, saying, "I am willing; be cleansed." Immediately his leprosy was cleansed.*

Matthew 8:16

> *When evening had come, they brought to Him many who were demon-possessed. And He cast out the spirits with a word, and healed all who were sick....*

Matthew 9:35

> *Then Jesus went about all the cities and villages, teaching in their synagogues, preaching the gospel of the kingdom, and healing every sickness and every disease among the people...*

Matthew 10:8

> *Jesus sent them out and commanded them saying...*"*Heal the sick, cleanse the lepers, cast out demons. Freely you have received, freely give.*

Matthew 12:13

> *Then He said to the man, "Stretch out your hand." And he stretched it out, and it was restored as whole as the other.*

Matthew 12:22

> *Then one was brought to Him who was demon-possessed, blind and mute; and He healed him, so that the blind and mute man both spoke and saw.*

Matthew 14:36

> *And begged Him that they might only touch the hem of His garment. And as many as touched it were made perfectly well.*

Matthew 15:30

> *Then great multitudes came to Him, having with them the lame, blind, mute, maimed, and many others; and they laid them down at Jesus' feet, and He healed them.*

Matthew 17:18

> *And Jesus rebuked the demon, and it came out of him; and the child was cured from that very hour.*

Matthew 19:2

> *And great multitudes followed Him, and He healed them there.*

Matthew 21:14

> *Then the blind and the lame came to Him in the temple, and He healed them.*

Mark 1:31

> *So He came and took her by the hand and lifted her up, and immediately the fever left her.*

Mark 10:52

> *Then Jesus said to him, "Go your way; your faith has made you well." And immediately he received his sight and followed Jesus on the road.*

Luke 7:21

> *And that very hour He cured many of infirmities, afflictions, and evil spirits; and to many blind He gave sight.*

Luke 13:13

> *And He laid His hands on her, and immediately she was made straight, and glorified GOD.*

Luke 17:14

> *So when He saw them, He said to them, "Go, show yourselves to the priests." And so it was that as they went they were cleansed.*

Luke 22:51

> *But Jesus answered and said, "Permit even this." And He touched his ear and healed him.*

John 4:50

> *Jesus said to him, "Go your way; your son lives." So the man believed the word that Jesus spoke to him, and he went his way.*

John 9:6,7

> *when He had said these things, He spat on the ground and made clay with the saliva; and He anointed the eyes of the blind man with clay. And He said to him, "Go wash in the pool of Siloam". So he went and washed, and came back seeing.*

James 5:16

> *...pray for one another that you may be healed.*

Isaiah 53:5

> *And by His stripes we are healed.*

Psalm 103:3

> *Who heals all your diseases.*

Acts 9:34

> *And Peter said to him, "Aeneas, Jesus the Christ heals you. Arise and make your bed." Then he arose immediately.*

I am certain that the gift of healing has been bestowed upon some of Christ's believers. They have been given the power to heal all manner of sickness and disease through the name of Jesus Christ. The healing may be that of a quieting spirit in times of great despair; the illumination of one's spirit when you pray; the reassurance that you receive when others are lifting you up in prayer, and the actual physical healing of a disease with the departing of infirmities or the removal of an evil or ungodly spirit or mind within a man.

"Heal me, O Lord and I shall be healed; save me and I shall be saved for thou art my praise" (*Jeremiah 17:14*)
I pray for the faith and hope and healing of all of you who are planning to win the fight against the disease of breast cancer.

Father, through your Son Jesus Christ in the Holy Spirit, we thank you for all the blessings that you have given us in our life, and we thank you for never giving up on us. We thank you for the love you have given us, and the sacrifice of your Son Jesus who died for our sins on the cross.

We confess that we are sinners and that we have sinned in our thoughts and words and in what we have done and what we have neglected to do, Do not hold our offenses against us but wash them away with the blood of Jesus Christ.

Father, grant that each breast cancer patient may be healed by you today through their faith in you. Grant each healing according to your will. Let all cancer be removed within the breast or any other part of their bodies. In the name of Jesus Christ I rebuke all cancer and every other sickness or disease in their bodies. Father may they through the power of Jesus Christ be healed and made whole.

Father, I know that you always hear and answer my prayer and that through you all things are possible. Bless and prosper each and everyone of them in all things and grant them perfect health and Your saving grace. Hold them close to you now and forever. Amen.

References:

1. Larsson, SC et al, Multiple Vitamins and Breast Cancer Risk, American Journal of Clinical Nutrition, Online March 24, 2010.
2. Larsson et al, *Am J Clin Nutr.* 2010;91:1268-1272. Abstract.
3. Moertel CG, Fleming TR, Rubin J, et al. A clinical trial of amygdalin (Laetrile) in the treatment of human cancer. N Engl J Med 1982;306:201–206.
4. Natural killer cells and lymphocytes increase in women with

breast cancer following massage therapy, Touch Research Institutes, University of Miami School of Medicine.

5. Mortimer P.A., Bates D.O., Brassington H.D. (1996) 'The prevalence of arm edema following treatment for breast cancer'. QJM, 89: 377-380.

6. Clark B., Sitzia J., Harlow W. (2005) 'Incidence and risk of arm edema following treatment for breast cancer: a three year follow-up study'. QJ Med, 98: 343-8.

7. Stein, R., Exercise Can Cut Risk of Dying From Breast Cancer, Washington Post, Wednesday, May 25, 2005

8. Del Giudice ME, Fantus IG, Ezzat S, et al: Insulin and related factors in premenopausal breast cancer risk. *Breast Cancer Res Treat* 47:111-120, 1998.

9. Irwin ML, Varma K, Alvarez-Reeves M, et al: Randomized controlled trial of aerobic exercise on insulin and insulin-like growth factors in breast cancer survivors: The Yale Exercise and Survivorship study. *Cancer Epidemiol Biomarkers Prev* 18:306-313, 2009.

10. Jermiah,D., Et al. Invasion of Other Gods, Word Publishing, 1995, p 29-35.

11. ClinicalTrials.gov Identifier: NCT00508794, Study ID Numbers: 2005-0522.

12. Rubinstein MP et al, IL-7 and IL-15 differentially regulate CD8+ T-cell subsets during contraction of the immune response., Blood, 2008,Vol: 112:9, p 3704-12.

13. von Mensdorff-Pouilly S, Verstraeten AA, Kenemans P, Snijdewint FG, Kok A, Van Kamp GJ, Paul MA, Van Diest PJ, Meijer S, Hilgers J: Survival in early breast cancer patients is favorably influenced by a natural humoral immune response to polymorphic epithelial mucin. J Clin Oncol 2000, 18:574-583

PERSONAL BREAST CANCER JOURNAL

A Record for Life and Health

for

_____

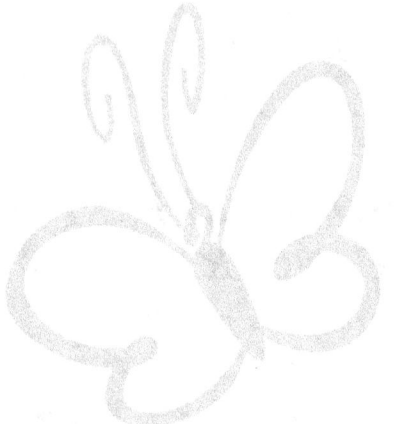

Family Member	Health Status	Cancer	Arthritis	Diabetes	Heart Disease	Lung Disease	Mental Illness
Father							
Mother							
Siblings							
Grand parents							
Children							

PERSONAL MEDICAL HISTORY

Name:

                      Sex:

Date of Birth:

Address:

Home Phone: *Work Phone:*

Mobile: *Email:*

Health Insurance
Carrier name and Address:
Group number:
Subscriber number:

Secondary Carrier Name and Address:
Group umber:
Subscriber number:

Doctor(s) Name   *Phone Number(s)*   *Address*

Current Medications   *Medications Allergies*

Food Allergies   *Other Allergies*

Date   *Previous Illnesses*   *Previous Surgeries*

Medication Name	Medical Condition	Start Date	End Date	Dosage

Medication Name	Medical Condition	Start Date	End Date	Dosage

QUESTIONS FOR YOUR PHYSICIANS

1. What is the stage of my breast cancer?
2. Could you go over the pathology report with me and may I have a copy of it and other pertinent report for my personal file?
3. What is the hormonal status of my tumor, ER, PR and Her2neu?
4. Am I a candidate for hormonal therapy?
5. What are my treatment options?
6. What are my surgery options for breast conservation?
7. Do I need a mastectomy or a lumpectomy?
8. Will I have an axillary node dissection or a sentinel node biopsy and what are the advantages and disadvantages of each?
9. Would you recommend reconstruction?
10. How does the reconstructed breast compare with the normal breast?
11. What are the limitations of reconstruction?
12. Will reconstruction interfere with radiation and chemotherapy treatments?
13. Will reconstruction interfere will my follow up exams?
14. Can I see photographs of cases you have reconstructed?
15. Do I need chemotherapy and/or radiation therapy?
16. What drugs will I be taking, the dosage and how ofter?
17. How long will chemotherapy last?
18. Will I be able to continue work while I receive treatment?
19. What side effects should I expect with chemotherapy and/or radiation therapy?
20. What would happen if I refuse treatment?
21. What types of complications may happen?
22. Based on my history should I and other members of my family be tested for the Breast cancer gene (BRCA1/BRCA2) and other genetic tests?
23. Do you have any suggestions for complementary alternative treatments or supplements?

24. What diet recommendations do you have?
25. Are there any local support groups for patients with breast cancer?

QUESTIONS JUST FOR YOU!

1. *How did you feel when you received the diagnosis of breast cancer and about what you were told?*
2. *Do you have a friend that you can talk to?*
3. *Are local support groups available?*
4. *What are your fears?*
5. *How do you feel about life and death?*
6. *What emotions have you experienced?*
7. *How well do you sleep?*
8. *Are you eating well?*
9. *Are you depressed?*
10. *Have you spoke to people in your church?*
11. *How do you relieve your stress?*
12. *How do you plan to cope with the disease?*
13. *Are you going to let family members, co-workers and friends know that you have the disease?*
14. *How do I feel about being a woman?*
15. *How has this diagnosis affected your sexuality?*
16. *How do I feel about the treatment recommended for you?*
17. *How do you feel about breast sparing surgery and mastectomy?*
18. *How will you cope if you have to lose your breast?*
19. *How do you feel about breast reconstruction?*
20. *How do you feel about chemotherapy?*
21. *What do you feel about losing your hair?*
22. *How has chemotherapy affected you and what changes have you made to cope with the treatment?*
23. *How do you feel about radiation therapy and how has it affected you?*
24. *How has anti-estrogen hormonal therapy affected you and what are you doing about the "Hot Flashes"?*
25. *What are your thoughts about complementary alter native therapies and which ones has you chosen to have?*
26. *How has this disease affected your relationship with your spouse or significant friend?*
27. *Do you have problems with intimacy?*

28. *If you are single, do you think you will still be able to date again or even find a spouse?*
29. *What do you feel about your health care team?*
30. *Has your family life changed, if so in what way?*
31. *Do people treat you differently?*
32. *How have members of your family been affected?*
33. *Has the support been there for you during your treatment?*
34. *What would you change about the treatment decisions that you have made?*
35. *Has your diet changed?*
36. *What steps are you making to keep healthy?*
37. *How do you feel about your general health?*
38. *What are your regrets about this entire experience?*
39. *How do you feel about the entire experience?*
40. *What are you planning for the rest of your life?*
41. *What are your short term and long term goals in life?*
42. *Has this experience brought you closer to God?*

MY LIVING WITH BREAST CANCER!

DATE

MY LIVING WITH BREAST CANCER!

DATE

MY LIVING WITH BREAST CANCER!

DATE

MY LIVING WITH BREAST CANCER!

DATE

296

MY LIVING WITH BREAST CANCER!

DATE

*MY LIVING WITH BREAST
CANCER!*

DATE

MY LIVING WITH BREAST CANCER!

DATE

MY LIVING WITH BREAST CANCER!

DATE

300

MY LIVING WITH BREAST CANCER!

DATE

MY LIVING WITH BREAST CANCER!

DATE

302

MY LIVING WITH BREAST CANCER!

DATE

MY LIVING WITH BREAST CANCER!

DATE

304

MY LIVING WITH BREAST CANCER!

DATE

MY LIVING WITH BREAST CANCER!

DATE

MY LIVING WITH BREAST CANCER!

DATE

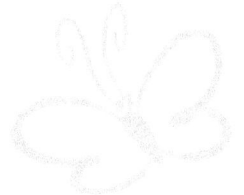

MY LIVING WITH BREAST CANCER!

DATE

308

MY LIVING WITH BREAST CANCER!

DATE

MY LIVING WITH BREAST CANCER!

DATE

MY LIVING WITH BREAST CANCER!

DATE

*MY LIVING WITH BREAST
CANCER!*

DATE

MY LIVING WITH BREAST CANCER!

DATE

MY LIVING WITH BREAST CANCER!

DATE

MY LIVING WITH BREAST CANCER!

DATE

MY LIVING WITH BREAST CANCER!

DATE

MY LIVING WITH BREAST CANCER!

DATE

MY LIVING WITH BREAST CANCER!

DATE

MY LIVING WITH BREAST CANCER!

DATE

MY LIVING WITH BREAST CANCER!

DATE

MY LIVING WITH BREAST CANCER!

DATE

MY LIVING WITH BREAST CANCER!

DATE

322

MY LIVING WITH BREAST CANCER!

DATE